Preface

300 Vocabulary for Nursing Career

"This is vocabulary words for nurses use in hospital"

This book is a collection of English vocabulary in the work category for nurses and doctors that are used in hospitals and communication in the general public health system and is suitable for anyone interested in medicine, nursing, and students who are beginning to learn nursing.

It would be a valuable resource for anyone interested in the medical field, especially those studying to become nurses or doctors. It could also be helpful for individuals looking to improve their understanding of medical terminology used in hospitals and public health settings. I'm sure readers will find it beneficial in expanding their vocabulary and knowledge related to medicine and nursing.

As they delve into the pages of this book, readers can expect to encounter a plethora of essential terms, phrases, and jargon commonly used in the healthcare industry. From medical procedures to patient care protocols, from anatomical terms to medication names, the book aims to provide a comprehensive overview of the vocabulary necessary for effective communication in the medical field. Whether you are a seasoned healthcare professional looking to brush up on your terminology or a newcomer eager to grasp the intricacies of nursing and medicine, this collection of English vocabulary promises to be a valuable asset in your journey towards mastering the language of healthcare.

Contents

25. Dementia

26. Dialysis

27. Diminished

28. Discharge

29. Diuretic

30. DNR (Do Not Resuscitate)

31. Dose

32. Drainage

33. Dyspnea

34. Edema

35. Electrocardiogram (EKG/ECG)

36. Electrolyte

37. Embolism

38. Endotracheal tube

39. Epinephrine

40. Erythema

41. Fecal

42. Fever

43. Foley catheter

44. Fracture

45. Gangrene

46. Gastrointestinal

47. Hematoma

48. Hemorrhage

49. Hospice

50. Hypertension

Page 53-151

51. Hypotension

52. Hypoxia

53. Incision

54. Infection

55. Inflammation

56. Infusion

57. Inpatient

58. IV (intravenous)

59. Isolation

60. Jaundice

61. Joint

62. Laceration

63. Larynx

64. Lavage

65. Lesion

66. Ligament

67. Lungs

68. Malnutrition

69. Malignant

70. Metastasis

71. Mucus

72. Myocardial infarction (MI)

73. Nasogastric tube

74. Nausea

75. Nebulizer

76. NPO (nothing by mouth)

77. Nutrients

78. Oncology

79. Ophthalmoscope

80. Orthopedic

81. Oxygen saturation

82. Pneumonia

83. Poisoning

84. Pulse

85. QD (once daily)

86. QID (four times daily)

87. Radiography

88. Respiration

89. Rehabilitation

90. Scalpel

91. Sepsis

92. Serology

93. Shock

94. Sore throat

95. Specimen

96. Stethoscope

97. Stool

98. Stroke

99. Subcutaneous

100. Surgery

101. Suture

102. Swab

103. Syringe

104. Tamponade

105. Telemetry

106. Thoracotomy

107. Tincture

108. Transfusion

109. Trauma

110. Triage

111. Ultrasound

112. Urinalysis

113. Vaccination

114. Vascular

115. Venipuncture

116. Ventilation

117. Vitals

118. Wound

119. X-ray

120. Yeast infection

121. Abdomen

122. Analgesic

123. Bronchoscopy

124. Carbuncle

125. CHF (congestive heart failure)

126. CPAP (continuous positive airway pressure)

127. CT scan (computed tomography)

128. Cyanosis

129. Dehydration

130. Diabetic

131. Diarrhea

132. Disinfection

133. Dorsal

134. Dystrophy

135. Echocardiogram

136. Edematous

137. Electroencephalogram (EEG)

138. Emesis

139. Emulsify

140. Febrile

141. Flatus

142. Gait

143. Hematocrit

144. Hemoglobin

145. Hemorrhoid

146. Hygiene

147. Immobilize

148. Impaired

149. Infarct

150. Ingest

151. Intake

152. Ischemia

153. Laryngitis

154. Lumbar puncture

155. Lymph nodes

156. Malignancy

157. Meningitis

158. Micturition

159. Myalgia

160. Nasal cannula

161. Necrosis

162. Neuropathy

163. Nystagmus

164. Ocular

165. Orthostatic

166. Otitis

167. Palliative

168. Paresthesia

169. Pathogen

170. Peritoneal

171. Pharyngitis

172. Pleura

173. Posterior

174. Prone

175. Protocol

176. Pruritus

177. PTP (prior to procedure)

178. Pulmonary embolism

179. Renal

180. Resuscitation

181. Rhinorrhea

182. Seizure

183. Sigmoidoscopy

184. Sinusitis

185. Sputum

186. Sterilization

187. Suppository

188. Syncope

189. Tachycardia

190. Thrombosis

191. Tidal volume

192. Topical

193. Tourniquet

194. Toxin

195. Tube feeding

196. Tumor

197. Ultrasonography

198. Urethra

199. Urology

200. Varicella

Page 151-211

201. Void

202. Vomiting

203. Waist circumference

204. Wheezing

205. Abscess

206. Active range of motion (AROM)

207. Adjuvant

208. Afebrile

209. Agglutination

210. Alopecia

211. Anaphylaxis
212. Angina
213. Anti-inflammatory
214. Apnea
215. Arrhythmia
216. Arterial
217. Atelectasis
218. Axilla
219. Benign
220. Biohazard
221. Bradycardia
222. Bronchitis
223. Budding
224. Carcinoma
225. Cardiopulmonary
226. Chemotherapy
227. Clotting
228. Colitis
229. Consciousness
230. Contracture
231. CPM (continuous passive motion)
232. Cystic fibrosis
233. Decubitus
234. Delirium
235. Disinfectant
236. Distension
237. Diurese
238. Dorsiflexion
239. Dysphagia
240. Edentulous
241. Endoscopy
242. Erythrocyte

243. Essential oils

244. Excretion

245. Expectorate

246. Fasting

247. Fistula

248. Gentian violet

249. Geriatric

250. Granulation

251. Hemostasis

252. Hyperglycemia

253. Hypoglycemia

254. Ileostomy

255. Induration

256. Ingestion

257. Inguinal

258. Inotropic

259. Iontophoresis

260. Irrigate

261. Keloid

262. Ketones

263. Liposuction

264. Lumpectomy

265. Lymphatic

266. Macular degeneration

267. Mammogram

268. Mastectomy

269. Melanoma

270. MRSA (methicillin-resistant Staphylococcus aureus)

271. Nasoenteric

272. Neuralgia

273. NSAID (non-steroidal anti-inflammatory drug)

274. Omentum

275. Ophthalmologist

276. Osteoporosis

277. Oxygen therapy

278. Pap smear

279. Paraplegia

280. Parkinson's disease

281. Paronychia

282. Peak flow

283. Perfusion

284. Perineal

285. Peritoneum

286. Phototherapy

287. Placenta

288. Pneumothorax

289. Polyps

290. Postoperative

291. Prosthesis

292. Ptosis

293. Quadriplegia

294. Reflexes

295. Regurgitation

296. Rhonchi

297. Serotonin

298. Sickle cell anemia

299. Stasis

300. Tonicity

Introduction

Welcome to "300 Vocabulary for Nursing Career" For these words nurses use in hospitals or for Medical and Nursing Terminology: A Comprehensive Guide".

This book is designed to provide a collection of essential vocabulary for individuals aspiring to become doctors and nurses. The terms included in this book are commonly used in hospitals and healthcare settings worldwide, making it a valuable resource for those looking to enter the medical profession.

Each term in this book will be carefully described and explained in the context of nursing and medical practice. By familiarizing yourself with these terms, you will develop a better understanding of the language used in healthcare, ultimately enhancing your ability to communicate effectively with colleagues and patients.

Whether you are a student embarking on your medical or nursing journey or a seasoned professional looking to expand your knowledge, this book is a valuable tool to help you navigate the complex world of healthcare terminology. Let's begin our exploration of the essential vocabulary used in the medical and nursing professions.

300 vocabulary words for nurses use in hospitals

1. Acuity

Acuity in nursing refers to the measure of the complexity and intensity of care required by patients in a healthcare setting. It is used to determine the level of staffing and resources needed to appropriately care for patients. Acuity is assessed based on various factors such as the severity of illness, the need for monitoring, the level of care required, and the amount of assistance needed with activities of daily living. Nursing acuity is often measured using standardized scoring systems to ensure that the appropriate level of care is provided to each patient.

2. Admit

In nursing, admit refers to the process of admitting a patient into a healthcare facility, such as a hospital or clinic. When a patient is admitted, it means that they are officially registered as a patient of the facility and are receiving care and treatment. The admission process typically involves gathering initial patient information, performing assessments, obtaining consent for treatment, and providing the patient with important information regarding their stay, such as their room assignment, healthcare team, and any necessary tests or procedures. Admitting a patient is an important step in organizing and coordinating their care within the healthcare facility.

3. Ambulate

In nursing, ambulation refers to the act of assisting or encouraging a patient to walk or move around. Ambulation is an essential component of patient care, as it helps patients maintain their mobility and prevent complications associated with immobility, such as muscle weakness, pressure ulcers, and blood clots. Nurses and other healthcare professionals may assist patients with ambulation if they are unable to walk independently or require additional support due to factors like injury, surgery, or weakness. Ambulation may involve helping a patient get out of bed, walking with them in the hallway, or providing assistance during physical therapy sessions. It is an important aspect of promoting patient independence and facilitating their recovery and rehabilitation.

4. Anesthesia

In nursing, anesthesia refers to the administration of medications or other substances that induce a temporary loss of sensation or consciousness. The purpose of anesthesia is to allow patients to undergo medical procedures or surgeries without experiencing pain or discomfort. Anesthesia is typically administered by an anesthesiologist, a specialized healthcare professional, or in some cases, by nurse anesthetists under the supervision of an anesthesiologist.

There are different types of anesthesia, including general anesthesia, regional anesthesia, and local anesthesia. General anesthesia involves inducing a state of unconsciousness, where the patient is asleep and does not feel any pain. Regional anesthesia involves numbing a specific region of the body, such as the lower half of the body (epidural anesthesia) or just an arm or leg (nerve block anesthesia). Local anesthesia numbs a small area of the body, such as a specific surgical site, and the patient remains awake. Nurses play a critical role in the administration and monitoring of anesthesia. They assist the anesthesia provider during the procedure, monitor the patient's vital signs, provide post-anesthesia care, and ensure the patient's safety and comfort throughout the process.

5. Antibiotic

In nursing, antibiotics refer to medications or substances that are used to treat bacterial infections. Antibiotics work by targeting and killing or inhibiting the growth of bacteria that cause infections. They are prescribed by healthcare providers when there is evidence or suspicion of a bacterial infection.

Nurses play a vital role in the administration and management of antibiotics. They ensure that antibiotics are administered at the prescribed dose, time, and route specified by the healthcare provider. Nurses also monitor the patient's response to the antibiotic therapy, which includes assessing for any side effects or adverse reactions. Additionally, nurses educate patients about the importance of completing the full course of antibiotics as prescribed, even if they start feeling better, to prevent the development of antibiotic resistance.

It is crucial for nurses to have knowledge about different antibiotics, including their mechanisms of action, indications, contraindications, and potential side effects. This allows nurses to provide safe and effective care to patients receiving antibiotic therapy.

6. Anticoagulant

In nursing, an anticoagulant refers to a medication that slows down or prevents blood clotting. These drugs are commonly used to treat or prevent blood clot formation in various medical conditions such as deep vein thrombosis, atrial fibrillation, pulmonary embolism, and heart attacks. Anticoagulants work by inhibiting certain clotting factors or enzymes that play a role in the coagulation process, helping to prevent the formation of dangerous blood clots that can obstruct blood vessels and cause serious complications. Nurses play a crucial role in administering and monitoring anticoagulant therapy, including assessing a patient's bleeding risk, monitoring blood coagulation levels, providing patient education on the medication's side effects and precautions, and ensuring appropriate dosage and timing for administration. Regular monitoring of anticoagulation is necessary to maintain therapeutic levels and minimize the risk of bleeding or clotting complications.

7. Antidepressant

In nursing, an antidepressant refers to a medication used to treat psychiatric conditions such as depression, anxiety disorders, obsessive-compulsive disorder, post-traumatic stress disorder, and other mood disorders. These drugs work by altering the balance of certain chemicals in the brain, such as serotonin, norepinephrine, and dopamine, which are involved in regulating mood, emotions, and mental well-being. Antidepressants are prescribed and managed by healthcare professionals, including nurses, in collaboration with psychiatrists or other mental health providers. Nurses play a critical role in assessing patients for mental health concerns, monitoring the effectiveness and side effects of antidepressant therapy, and providing education and support to patients and their families regarding proper medication use, potential interactions, and potential symptoms to watch for. They may also work alongside other members of the healthcare team to develop comprehensive treatment plans that may include counseling, therapy, and other interventions in addition to medication management.

8. Aseptic

In nursing, the term "aseptic" refers to practices and techniques that prevent the introduction, growth, and spread of microorganisms (such as bacteria, viruses, and fungi) that may cause infections. Aseptic techniques are necessary to create and maintain a sterile or clean environment, especially in healthcare settings such as hospitals, operating rooms, and clinics.

Nurses follow aseptic principles to minimize the risk of infections during procedures, surgeries, wound care, and the administration of medications or intravenous fluids. Examples of aseptic techniques include:

1. Hand hygiene: Strict handwashing or the use of alcohol-based hand sanitizers before and after patient care activities.

2. Use of personal protective equipment (PPE): Wearing gloves, masks, gowns, and goggles or face shields to protect both the healthcare worker and the patient from the transmission of microorganisms.

3. Sterile technique: Following specific protocols for preparing and handling sterile equipment, instruments, dressings, or solutions to prevent contamination.

4. Proper disinfection and cleaning: Using appropriate disinfectants and cleaning agents to ensure surfaces, medical equipment, and patient care areas are free from harmful microorganisms.

5. Safe injection practices: Utilizing sterile needles, syringes, and vials, and adhering to guidelines for proper disposal of sharps and contaminated materials.

By practicing aseptic techniques, nurses contribute to the prevention of healthcare-associated infections and promote patient safety and well-being.

9. Auscultate

In nursing, auscultation refers to the act of listening to sounds produced by the body using a stethoscope. It is a commonly used technique to assess and gather information about the functioning of various organ systems, particularly the cardiovascular and respiratory systems.

During auscultation, nurses place the stethoscope on specific areas of the body to listen to internal sounds. For example:

1. Cardiovascular auscultation involves listening to heart sounds such as the lub-dub sound of the heart valves, abnormal heart murmurs, or irregular rhythms.

2. Respiratory auscultation involves listening to breath sounds in different areas of the lungs to assess air movement, detect abnormal sounds (such as crackles, wheezes, or rhonchi), or monitor respiratory patterns.

Auscultation is also used in other areas of nursing care, such as assessing bowel sounds in the abdomen or assessing sounds in the arteries for signs of vascular abnormalities or narrowing.

Nurses are trained to identify normal and abnormal sounds during auscultation, which can provide valuable diagnostic information to aid in the evaluation, treatment, and monitoring of patients. It is a non-invasive and cost-effective assessment technique that is widely utilized in routine nursing assessments as well as in more critical situations.

10. Autonomy

In nursing, autonomy refers to a patient's right to make their own decisions about their healthcare and participate actively in their treatment plan. It is one of the fundamental ethical principles in healthcare, referred to as patient autonomy or individual autonomy.

Autonomy emphasizes the respect for a patient's self-determination and their ability to make choices according to their own values, beliefs, and preferences. Nurses play a crucial role in promoting and safeguarding patient autonomy by:

1. Providing accurate and reliable information: Nurses educate patients about their health condition, available treatment options, risks, benefits, and alternatives. They ensure that patients have the necessary information to make informed decisions about their care.

2. Facilitating shared decision-making: Nurses collaborate with patients, their families, and other healthcare professionals in the decision-making process. They engage in open and respectful communication, actively listen to patients' concerns and preferences, and support them in making decisions that align with their values and goals.

3. Respecting patient choices: Nurses respect and honor the decisions made by competent patients, even if they may not necessarily agree with them. They advocate for their patients' choices, ensuring that their decisions are reflected in their care plans and treatment options.

4. Protecting patient rights: Nurses ensure that patients' rights to autonomy are upheld and protected. This includes privacy and confidentiality, informed consent, and the right to refuse or discontinue treatment.

5. Providing patient education: Nurses empower patients by providing education and resources to enhance their understanding of their health conditions, treatment options, and self-care management. This allows patients to actively participate in their healthcare decisions and take ownership of their well-being.

Overall, autonomy in nursing recognizes and promotes the importance of patient-centered care, respecting patients' rights, and involving them in decision-making processes to achieve the best possible outcomes.

11. Bacterium

Bacterium refers to a single bacterium, which is a microscopic organism that can cause infection or disease in humans. In nursing, understanding bacterium is important for infection control measures, proper sterilization techniques, and recommending appropriate antibiotic treatments. Nurses need to be knowledgeable about various bacteria and their characteristics in order to provide effective care and prevent the spread of infections in healthcare settings.

12. Bandage

A bandage in nursing refers to a material or dressing used to cover a wound or injury. It is an essential component of wound care and is employed to protect the wound, promote healing, prevent infection, and provide support. Bandages can be made of various materials such as cloth, gauze, adhesive, or elastic. They can be applied in different ways, depending on the type and location of the wound. Nurses are trained in proper bandage techniques to ensure the safety and comfort of the patient, as well as to facilitate healing and prevent complications.

13. Bedpan

A bedpan in nursing refers to a shallow, flat-bottomed container designed to be placed under a patient's buttocks to collect urine or feces while they are unable to use the toilet. Bedpans are commonly used in healthcare settings for patients who are bedridden, have limited mobility, or are unable to get out of bed due to a medical condition, injury, or post-surgical recovery. They are made of plastic or metal and have a low rim to provide comfort and ease of use. Nurses assist patients with using a bedpan, ensuring privacy, maintaining cleanliness, and providing appropriate hygiene care after its use.

14. Blood pressure

Blood pressure in nursing refers to the measurement of the force of blood against the walls of the arteries as the heart pumps it around the body. It is an important vital sign that provides information about a person's cardiovascular health. Blood pressure is measured using a sphygmomanometer, which consists of an inflatable cuff and a pressure gauge. The measurement is expressed as two values: systolic pressure over diastolic pressure, for example, 120/80 mmHg. Systolic pressure represents the force when the heart contracts and pumps blood, while diastolic pressure represents the force when the heart is at rest between beats. Nurses are responsible for monitoring patients' blood pressure regularly, both in clinical settings and during home visits, as it helps to detect hypertension or hypotension, assess treatment effectiveness, and evaluate overall cardiovascular health. Nurses also educate patients on maintaining healthy blood pressure levels and managing any blood pressure related conditions.

15. Catheter

A catheter in nursing refers to a medical device that is used to introduce or withdraw fluids from the body. It is a flexible tube that is inserted into a specific area, such as a blood vessel, bladder, or vein, to perform various medical procedures. Catheters are made from different materials, depending on their purpose and location of insertion.

In nursing, catheters are commonly used for different purposes such as:

- Urinary catheters: These are inserted into the bladder through the urethra to drain urine in patients who may be unable to urinate on their own, such as those with urinary retention or undergoing surgery.
- Intravenous catheters: These are inserted into a vein and used for delivering medications, fluids, or blood products directly into the bloodstream.
- Central venous catheters: These are long, flexible tubes inserted into large veins near the heart, typically used for delivering medications, nutrition, or hemodialysis over a prolonged period.
- Arterial catheters: These are inserted into an artery for continuous monitoring of blood pressure and arterial blood gases.
- Cardiac catheters: These are inserted into blood vessels in the heart for diagnostic purposes or to perform interventional procedures such as angioplasty or stent placement.

Nurses play a crucial role in the proper insertion, care, and removal of catheters to maintain aseptic technique, prevent infections, and ensure patient comfort and safety. They also monitor patients for any complications associated with catheter use and provide education on catheter care and hygiene.

16. Central line

A central line in nursing refers to a type of intravenous (IV) access device that is inserted into a large vein in the body for various medical purposes. Also known as a central venous catheter (CVC), it is typically placed in veins near the heart, such as the subclavian vein or the jugular vein.

Unlike regular IV lines, which are inserted into peripheral veins in the arms or hands, a central line provides access to larger veins and is used for more complex medical treatments. It allows for the administration of medications, fluids, blood products, and nutritional support, as well as the monitoring of central venous pressure.

The insertion of a central line is a sterile procedure performed by trained healthcare professionals, often under ultrasound guidance. Nurses play a key role in the care and management of central lines, including dressing changes, monitoring for signs of infection or complications, and ensuring proper functioning and maintenance.

Central lines may be used in various clinical settings, including intensive care units, operating rooms, and certain outpatient settings. They are commonly used for patients who require long-term IV therapy, frequent blood draws, or specialized treatments such as chemotherapy or hemodialysis. However, central lines carry a risk of complications, such as infection and thrombosis, so proper care and monitoring are essential to minimize these risks.

17. Cervix

In nursing, the cervix refers to the lower narrow portion of the uterus that connects it to the vagina. It is a cylindrical structure composed of fibrous tissue and muscle, with an opening at the center known as the cervical os. The cervix plays a crucial role in reproductive health, as it allows for the passage of menstrual blood from the uterus and serves as the entrance to the uterus during sexual intercourse and childbirth.

In the context of nursing, the cervix is an important anatomical structure that nurses may assess and monitor in various situations, including:

1. Gynecological exams: Nurses may assist healthcare providers during pelvic exams to assess the health of the cervix, which may involve visual inspection, palpation, or the use of specialized instruments like a speculum.

2. Pap smears: Nurses may perform or assist with pap smears, which involve collecting cells from the cervix to screen for cervical cancer or abnormalities.

3. Labor and delivery: During childbirth, nurses may monitor the dilation and effacement (thinning) of the cervix to assess the progress of labor. They may also perform cervical checks to determine if a woman is in the active phase of labor.

4. Cervical ripening: In certain situations, such as induction of labor, nurses may be involved in the administration or management of medications or procedures to help ripen or dilate the cervix in preparation for childbirth.

Understanding the anatomy and function of the cervix is essential for nurses to provide comprehensive care related to women's health, including preventive screenings, reproductive health education, and support during labor and delivery.

18. Circulation

Circulation in nursing refers to the movement of blood through the body's blood vessels, which is essential for delivering oxygen and nutrients to various body tissues and removing waste products. Nurses play a crucial role in assessing and monitoring a patient's circulatory system by checking vital signs, such as heart rate, blood pressure, and oxygen levels, as well as observing for any signs of impaired circulation, such as cool or pale skin, weak or absent pulses, or edema. Nurses also provide interventions to promote proper circulation, such as positioning patients correctly, administering medications, or managing intravenous fluids.

19. Colostomy

Colostomy in nursing refers to a surgical procedure that involves creating an opening in the abdominal wall, called a stoma, through which a portion of the colon (large intestine) is brought to the surface. This procedure is typically done when a portion of the colon needs to be bypassed or removed due to various medical conditions, such as colorectal cancer, inflammatory bowel disease, or intestinal obstruction.

In nursing, the care of patients with a colostomy involves providing education and support to help them adjust to life with a stoma. Nurses teach patients how to care for their colostomy bags, which collect stool from the stoma. This includes proper cleaning, emptying, and changing of the bags. Nurses also monitor patients for any complications or issues related to the colostomy, such as infection, skin irritation, or blockage, and provide appropriate interventions. Additionally, they offer emotional support and education to help patients maintain their independence and quality of life with a colostomy.

20. Coma

Coma in nursing refers to a state of unconsciousness in which an individual is unresponsive and unable to be awakened. It is a severe medical condition that may be caused by various factors, such as traumatic brain injury, stroke, drug overdose, severe infection, metabolic disorders, or lack of oxygen to the brain.

In nursing, the care of patients in a coma involves close monitoring and assessment of their vital signs, neurological status, and overall condition. Nurses play a critical role in providing ongoing care to these patients, including the administration of medications, monitoring and maintaining ventilation, suctioning secretions, monitoring intracranial pressure if applicable, and preventing complications such as pressure ulcers and contractures.

Nurses also provide support and education to the patient's family, as they may be emotionally overwhelmed and require information on the patient's condition, prognosis, and treatment plan. Depending on the cause and severity of the coma, nursing care may focus on assisting patients in regaining consciousness or providing end-of-life care and comfort measures.

21. Contagious

In nursing, "contagious" refers to the ability of a disease or infection to be transmitted from one person to another through direct or indirect contact. When a disease or infection is contagious, it means that it can be spread easily from an infected individual to others who come into contact with them.

Nurses play a vital role in identifying and managing contagious conditions in healthcare settings. They follow strict infection control protocols to prevent the transmission of infectious diseases. This includes practicing proper hand hygiene, wearing personal protective equipment (such as gloves, masks, and gowns), and implementing isolation precautions when necessary. Nurses also educate patients, families, and visitors on the importance of infection prevention measures, such as covering the mouth when coughing or sneezing, properly disposing of tissues, and avoiding close contact with infected individuals.

Additionally, nurses closely monitor patients with contagious conditions to ensure they receive appropriate treatment, maintain isolation as needed, and observe for any worsening of symptoms or complications. By implementing infection control practices and providing comprehensive care, nurses help prevent the spread of contagious diseases and promote the health and safety of both patients and healthcare providers.

22. CPR

CPR in nursing stands for Cardiopulmonary Resuscitation. It is an emergency procedure performed to manually preserve brain function until further medical intervention can be administered, in cases of cardiac arrest or when a person's heart and/or breathing has stopped.

In CPR, nurses perform a combination of chest compressions and rescue breaths to help circulate oxygenated blood to vital organs, particularly the brain. The chest compressions are performed to manually pump the heart, mimicking its pumping action, while rescue breaths involve providing artificial ventilation by delivering breaths into the patient's airway to maintain oxygenation.

Nurses are trained in CPR techniques, which include proper hand placement, compression depth and rate, and the ratio of chest compressions to rescue breaths. They also learn to recognize the signs of a cardiac arrest and quickly initiate CPR when necessary.

Alongside CPR, nurses may use automated external defibrillators (AEDs) to deliver electrical shocks to the heart to restore normal rhythm. They also monitor vital signs and administer appropriate medications or interventions as directed by the medical team during resuscitation efforts.

Given their critical role in patient care, nurses are often at the frontline in initiating CPR and providing life-saving interventions, both within hospital and community settings.

23. Critical

In nursing, "critical" refers to the condition or situation in which a patient's health status is deteriorating rapidly and immediate intervention is required to prevent further harm or potential loss of life. Critical situations can arise in various healthcare settings, such as intensive care units (ICUs), emergency departments, or during specific procedures or treatments.

Nurses working in critical care or emergency settings are trained to assess and manage patients with complex and unstable conditions. They closely monitor vital signs, perform ongoing assessments, and use their clinical judgment to identify early signs of deterioration. When a patient becomes critical, nurses must act quickly and decisively to provide appropriate interventions, call for assistance from the healthcare team, and initiate lifesaving measures as necessary.

Critical nursing also involves the ability to prioritize care and multitask effectively. Nurses may be responsible for administering medications, titrating IV drips, managing ventilators, inserting invasive monitoring devices, and coordinating diagnostic tests or interventions. They work closely with other members of the healthcare team to develop and implement comprehensive care plans tailored to the patient's specific needs.

Furthermore, critical nursing requires excellent communication and collaboration skills to effectively communicate with patients, their families, and other healthcare professionals involved in the patient's care. Nurses must be able to provide clear and concise updates on the patient's condition, relay information in urgent situations, and advocate for the patient's best interests.

Overall, critical nursing involves the ability to respond swiftly and decisively to rapidly changing patient conditions, provide optimal care and interventions, and ensure the best possible outcomes for critically ill or injured patients.

24. Defibrillator

In nursing, a defibrillator refers to a medical device used to deliver an electrical shock to the heart when a person is experiencing a life-threatening cardiac rhythm disturbance, such as ventricular fibrillation or ventricular tachycardia. These arrhythmias can cause the heart to stop pumping effectively, leading to cardiac arrest.

Defibrillators are designed to restore the heart's normal rhythm by delivering a controlled electric shock to the chest wall. This shock interrupts the chaotic electrical activity in the heart, allowing the heart's natural pacemaker to reestablish a coordinated heartbeat.

Nurses play a critical role in the use of defibrillators in various healthcare settings, including hospitals, emergency departments, critical care units, and ambulatory care centers. They are trained in advanced cardiac life support (ACLS) and are responsible for recognizing life-threatening cardiac rhythms, determining when defibrillation is necessary, and administering the appropriate treatment.

Nurses assess the patient's condition and, if defibrillation is indicated, follow proper safety protocols, such as ensuring that everyone is clear of the patient before delivering the electric shock. They apply the defibrillator pads to the patient's chest, initiate the machine, and monitor the patient's response. Nurses also coordinate with the healthcare team to ensure that further interventions and care are promptly provided after defibrillation.

Moreover, nurses educate patients, families, and caregivers on the use and importance of defibrillators. They may provide instruction on how to use automated external defibrillators (AEDs) in public places or community settings, emphasizing the crucial role of early defibrillation in improving survival rates for sudden cardiac arrest.

25. Dementia

In nursing, dementia refers to a group of conditions characterized by a decline in cognitive function and memory, leading to impairment in activities of daily living and overall functioning. Dementia is not a specific disease but a syndrome encompassing a range of symptoms associated with the progressive decline of cognitive abilities.

Nurses play a significant role in the care of individuals with dementia. They provide assessment, support, and interventions to manage the physical, emotional, and social needs of patients with this condition. Nursing care for individuals with dementia includes:

1. Assessment: Nurses perform comprehensive assessments to evaluate the individual's cognitive status, functional abilities, behavioral changes, and overall health. They monitor and assess changes in cognition, behavior, and physical status over time.

2. Medication management: Nurses collaborate with healthcare providers to administer and monitor medications prescribed for managing dementia symptoms, such as memory-enhancing drugs or medications to address behavioral issues.

3. Personal care assistance: Nurses help individuals with dementia with activities of daily living, including bathing, dressing, toileting, and eating. They ensure that the environment is safe and supportive for the specific needs of individuals with dementia.

4. Communication and emotional support: Nurses employ effective communication techniques to interact and engage with individuals with dementia, using simple language, non-verbal cues, and patience. They provide emotional support to individuals and their families, as they navigate the challenging journey of dementia.

5. Collaborative care: Nurses work in collaboration with interdisciplinary healthcare teams, including physicians, social workers, occupational therapists, and speech therapists, to develop and implement individualized care plans for individuals with dementia.

Nurses also provide education and guidance to families and caregivers on how to effectively care for and communicate with individuals with dementia. They assist in developing strategies to manage behavior changes, promote a supportive environment, and engage individuals in meaningful activities to maintain their quality of life.

26. Dialysis

In nursing, dialysis refers to a medical procedure that helps perform the function of the kidneys when they are no longer able to adequately filter and remove waste products and excess fluid from the body. Dialysis is commonly used in the treatment of end-stage renal disease (ESRD) or acute kidney injury.

There are two primary types of dialysis: hemodialysis and peritoneal dialysis.

1. Hemodialysis: Hemodialysis involves the use of a machine called a dialyzer to filter the blood. During hemodialysis, blood is pumped from the patient's body through specialized tubing into the dialyzer, where it is cleaned and filtered. The filtered blood is then returned to the patient's body. Hemodialysis is typically performed in a dialysis center or hospital setting, and nurses play a crucial role in monitoring the patient's vital signs, ensuring proper dialysis machine functioning, and assessing for any complications or adverse reactions during and after the procedure. They also provide education regarding diet, fluid restrictions, medication management, and preventive care for patients on long-term hemodialysis.

2. Peritoneal dialysis: Peritoneal dialysis involves the use of the peritoneal membrane in the abdomen to remove waste and excess fluid from the body. A sterile dialysis

solution is introduced into the abdominal cavity through a catheter, and it is allowed to dwell for a specified period. The solution absorbs waste products and excess fluid, and then it is drained out of the body. Peritoneal dialysis can be performed at home or in a healthcare facility, and nurses are responsible for teaching patients and their caregivers how to perform the procedure, ensuring proper technique, and monitoring for any complications or infections.

Nurses also play a critical role in assessing and managing complications of dialysis, such as infection, vascular access issues, fluid imbalances, electrolyte abnormalities, and changes in the patient's overall condition. They collaborate with the healthcare team to provide comprehensive care, promote patient comfort, and optimize dialysis outcomes.

27. Diminished

In nursing, "diminished" refers to a decrease or reduction in a specific aspect or function related to a patient's health status. It implies that there has been a decline or impairment compared to what is considered normal or expected.

The term "diminished" is often used to describe various physical, cognitive, or sensory functions in healthcare settings. For example:

1. Diminished respiratory function: This refers to a decrease in the efficiency or capacity of the respiratory system, such as reduced lung function or impaired oxygenation. Nurses assess and monitor respiratory rates, oxygen saturation levels, and other respiratory parameters to identify any signs of diminished respiratory function.

2. Diminished mobility: This refers to a decreased ability to move or walk independently. It can occur as a result of various factors, including musculoskeletal problems, neurological conditions, or generalized weakness. Nurses assess and assist patients with impaired mobility, implement appropriate interventions, and

collaborate with other healthcare professionals to develop a plan of care that helps enhance mobility and prevent complications such as falls or pressure ulcers.

3. Diminished cognitive function: This refers to a decline in mental processes and abilities, including memory, attention, problem-solving, and decision-making skills. It can be seen in conditions such as dementia or delirium. Nurses conduct cognitive assessments, provide support and appropriate interventions, and collaborate with interdisciplinary teams to manage and improve cognitive functioning whenever feasible.

4. Diminished sensory perception: This refers to a reduction in the function of sensory organs, including sight, hearing, touch, taste, and smell. Nurses assess a patient's sensory perception and provide appropriate accommodations or interventions to compensate for any sensory deficits.

In nursing, recognizing and addressing areas of diminished function is crucial for providing appropriate care and interventions to enhance the patient's overall well-being and quality of life. Nurses work collaboratively with other healthcare professionals to develop comprehensive care plans that address the specific needs associated with diminished functions.

28. Discharge

In nursing, "discharge" refers to the process of releasing a patient from a healthcare facility, such as a hospital, clinic, or nursing home, after completing a course of treatment or receiving necessary care. It involves the coordination of various activities and tasks to ensure a smooth transition for the patient from the healthcare setting to their home or an appropriate care setting.

The discharge process in nursing typically involves the following components:

1. Education and instructions: Nurses provide patients and their caregivers with important information about the patient's condition, medications, follow-up appointments, and self-care instructions. This includes guidance on managing symptoms, wound care, medication administration, dietary restrictions, and any necessary medical equipment or supplies.

2. Medication management: Nurses review and reconcile the patient's medications, ensuring that they have a sufficient supply of prescribed medications and understanding how and when to take them. They may also arrange for home delivery of medications or coordinate with the patient's pharmacy.

3. Caregiver support: If the patient requires assistance from a caregiver at home, nurses provide education and support to the caregiver as appropriate. This includes teaching them how to perform specific tasks, such as administering medications, changing dressings, or assisting with mobility or personal care.

4. Discharge planning and coordination: Nurses collaborate with the healthcare team to develop an individualized discharge plan that addresses the patient's ongoing care needs. This may involve arranging for home health services, rehabilitation programs, medical equipment, or referrals to other healthcare providers or community resources. Nurses ensure that all necessary documentation and arrangements are made for post-discharge care.

5. Follow-up: Nurses schedule any required follow-up appointments with healthcare providers and provide the patient with the necessary information and reminders. They may also conduct phone or virtual follow-up assessments to monitor the patient's progress and address any concerns or questions.

The goal of the discharge process is to facilitate a safe and smooth transition for patients from the healthcare facility to their home or another appropriate care setting, with the necessary support and resources in place to continue their recovery and manage their healthcare needs.

29. Diuretic

In nursing, a diuretic refers to a medication that promotes diuresis, which is the increased production of urine by the kidneys. Diuretics work by increasing the excretion of sodium and water from the body, which can help reduce fluid retention and edema.

Diuretics are commonly prescribed for various medical conditions, including hypertension (high blood pressure), congestive heart failure, kidney disease, and certain types of edema. Nurses play a crucial role in administering and monitoring the effects of diuretic medications.

When administering diuretics, nurses need to monitor the patient's vital signs, including blood pressure, heart rate, and respiratory rate. They also assess the patient for any signs of dehydration, electrolyte imbalances, or adverse effects related to the medication.

Nurses educate patients about their diuretic medication, such as the importance of taking it as prescribed, the potential side effects, and the need for regular monitoring of fluid intake, weight, and urine output. Additionally, they provide guidance on maintaining a balanced diet, including foods rich in potassium, as some diuretics may cause potassium depletion.

Nurses collaborate with the healthcare team to assess and adjust the dosage of diuretics based on the patient's response and overall condition. They communicate any relevant changes in the patient's fluid balance, electrolyte levels, or symptoms to the healthcare team and work towards achieving optimal outcomes and medication effectiveness.

Overall, nurses in various healthcare settings, such as hospitals, clinics, and long-term care facilities, are responsible for administering diuretic medications, monitoring the patient's response and well-being, managing potential side effects, and providing patient education and support related to diuretic therapy.

30. DNR (Do Not Resuscitate)

In nursing, DNR (Do Not Resuscitate) refers to a legal order or directive that indicates a patient's wish to not undergo cardiopulmonary resuscitation (CPR) in the event of cardiac arrest or respiratory failure.

A DNR order is typically determined through discussions between the patient, family members or caregivers, and the healthcare team, including physicians and nurses. It is an important part of advance care planning and allows patients to make decisions about their end-of-life care.

Nurses play a crucial role in ensuring that a patient's wishes regarding resuscitation are honored. This includes:

1. Communication: Nurses facilitate conversations with patients, their families, and physicians to help clarify the patient's preferences and goals of care. They provide information about the potential outcomes of CPR, the benefits and risks, and alternative options for end-of-life care.

2. Documentation: Nurses ensure that the DNR order is properly documented in the patient's medical record and communicated to all members of the healthcare team involved in their care. The DNR order should be clearly visible and easily accessible to ensure compliance with the patient's wishes.

3. Education: Nurses educate patients, families, and caregivers about the implications of the DNR order, including the fact that it does not mean withdrawing all treatment or care. They explain that the focus shifts towards comfort, symptom management, and maintaining dignity at the end of life.

4. Advocacy: Nurses advocate for the patient's preferences and ensure that the DNR order is respected during care delivery. They communicate this information to other healthcare providers and assist in educating and supporting the patient's family members and caregivers.

It is essential for nurses to approach discussions about DNR orders with sensitivity, empathy, and respect for the patient's autonomy and values. They play a pivotal role in facilitating understanding, providing emotional support, and promoting shared decision-making during this challenging and sensitive aspect of end-of-life care.

31. Dose

In nursing, "dose" refers to the specific amount of medication or treatment prescribed to a patient at a given time. It represents the quantity of a medication or treatment that is administered to achieve the desired therapeutic effect.

Nurses play a vital role in ensuring the accurate administration of medication doses according to the healthcare provider's prescription. This involves several key responsibilities:

1. Calculation: Nurses calculate medication doses based on the healthcare provider's prescription and the specific form of the medication available (e.g., tablets, liquid, injectable). They carefully read and interpret the prescription and use mathematical calculations to determine the correct dosage.

2. Preparation: Nurses prepare medication dosages by accurately measuring or counting the specified amount of medication needed for administration. This may involve reconstituting powdered medications, drawing up medications from vials or ampules, or dividing tablets or capsules as necessary.

3. Administration: Nurses safely administer the correct dose of medication to the patient through various routes, such as oral, intravenous, intramuscular,

subcutaneous, or topical. They adhere to proper medication administration techniques and follow organizational policies and procedures for medication safety.

4. Documentation: Nurses document the medication dose administered, including the medication name, dosage, route, time, and any relevant patient responses or observations. Accurate and timely documentation is crucial for monitoring medication effectiveness, ensuring continuity of care, and minimizing the risk of medication errors.

Nurses also consider various factors when determining the appropriate dose for a patient, such as the patient's age, weight, renal or hepatic function, and any specific clinical considerations or contraindications. They vigilantly monitor the patient's response to medication, assessing for therapeutic effects, adverse reactions, or any changes in the patient's condition.

Additionally, nurses provide patient education regarding medication dosages, including the importance of taking the prescribed dose as directed, potential side effects or interactions, and the importance of adhering to the prescribed regimen.

Overall, accurate and safe medication dosing is a critical responsibility of nurses, ensuring that patients receive the appropriate amount of medication to achieve the desired therapeutic effect and promoting patient safety and well-being.

32. Drainage

In nursing, "drainage" refers to the fluid, pus, or other substances that are collected or discharged from a wound, body cavity, or surgical site. It can be an essential aspect of patient care, as it helps to remove unwanted fluids or substances, promote healing, and prevent infection.

Nurses play a vital role in managing and monitoring drainage in various healthcare settings. This involves several key responsibilities:

1. Assessment: Nurses assess the characteristics of the drainage, including color, consistency, amount, and odor. They also evaluate the site or wound for signs of infection, such as increased redness, swelling, warmth, or presence of pus.

2. Collection and measurement: Nurses collect and measure the drainage to monitor the amount and document changes over time. This may involve using wound dressings, drainage bags, or other specialized devices to collect the fluid. Accurate measurement is essential for tracking patient progress and assessing the effectiveness of treatment.

3. Documentation: Nurses document the characteristics and amount of drainage in the patient's medical record. This helps in communication among healthcare providers, tracking changes in the patient's condition, and ensuring continuity of care.

4. Management: Nurses are responsible for maintaining the cleanliness and integrity of drainage systems or dressings. They may need to change dressings, empty drainage bags, or clean the collection site in a sterile manner. Nurses also assess the patient's response to treatment and monitor for any signs of complications related to drainage, such as infection or excessive bleeding.

Additionally, nurses provide patient and family education regarding drainage management. They teach proper hygiene practices, signs of infection to watch for, and techniques for managing drainage devices or dressings at home if necessary.

By effectively managing drainage, nurses help prevent complications, promote wound healing, and ensure patient comfort. They collaborate with the healthcare team to develop individualized care plans that address the specific needs of each patient and strive to achieve optimal outcomes in drainage management.

33. Dyspnea

In nursing, "dyspnea" refers to the sensation of breathlessness or difficulty breathing. It is a subjective experience where a patient feels as though they cannot get enough air or are struggling to breathe adequately. Dyspnea can range in severity and may be caused by various underlying medical conditions or factors.

Nurses play a critical role in assessing and managing dyspnea in patients. This involves several key responsibilities:

1. Assessment: Nurses assess the patient's breathing pattern, respiratory rate, lung sounds, oxygen saturation levels, and overall respiratory effort. They ask the patient about their subjective experience of breathlessness, such as the intensity, duration, and any precipitating factors. Nurses also gather information about any underlying conditions or triggers that may contribute to dyspnea.

2. Monitoring: Nurses continuously monitor the patient's respiratory status and vital signs, paying particular attention to signs of respiratory distress or worsening dyspnea. They assess and document the effectiveness of any interventions implemented to alleviate the dyspnea.

3. Collaboration: Nurses collaborate with the healthcare team, including physicians, respiratory therapists, and other healthcare professionals, to determine the underlying cause of dyspnea and develop an appropriate plan of care. This may involve diagnostic tests, medication adjustments, or other interventions as indicated.

4. Interventions: Nurses implement interventions to manage and alleviate dyspnea, based on the underlying cause and the patient's specific needs. This may include administering oxygen therapy, positioning the patient in a comfortable and supportive position, providing breathing exercises, administering medications, or assisting with coughing or effective airway clearance.

5. Education and support: Nurses provide patient and family education on dyspnea management techniques, self-monitoring, and when to seek medical attention. They also offer emotional support and reassurance to help alleviate anxiety and distress associated with dyspnea.

Prompt identification and management of dyspnea are crucial to ensure the patient's comfort and well-being. Nurses use their clinical skills and expertise to assess, intervene, and advocate for the patient to effectively manage dyspnea and collaborate with the healthcare team to address its underlying causes.

34. Edema

In nursing, "edema" refers to the abnormal accumulation of fluid in body tissues, resulting in swelling. It occurs when there is an imbalance in the movement of fluid between the blood vessels and the surrounding tissues. Edema can affect various parts of the body, including the legs, ankles, feet, hands, face, and abdomen.

Nurses play a crucial role in assessing and managing edema in patients. This involves several key responsibilities:

1. Assessment: Nurses assess the extent and location of the edema, as well as any contributing factors or underlying conditions. They evaluate the consistency, symmetry, and degree of swelling, and any associated changes in skin color or texture. Nurses also assess the patient's vital signs, weight, and any signs of respiratory distress or other symptoms associated with fluid overload.

2. Documentation: Nurses accurately document the assessment findings related to edema, including the location, severity, and any associated symptoms. This documentation helps track changes in edema over time and communicate important information to the healthcare team.

3. Treatment and management: Nurses implement appropriate interventions to manage edema based on the underlying cause and the patient's overall condition. This may include elevation of the affected limbs, compression therapy, dietary modifications (such as reducing sodium intake), use of diuretic medications to promote fluid excretion, and other measures to facilitate fluid balance and enhance circulation.

4. Education: Nurses provide patient education on measures to manage and prevent edema. This may include guidance on self-care techniques, such as elevating legs, wearing compression stockings or garments, regular physical activity, and adhering to medication regimens. Nurses also provide education to patients and families about recognizing signs of worsening edema and when to seek medical attention.

5. Collaboration: Nurses collaborate with the healthcare team to identify and address underlying causes of edema. This may involve consultations with physicians, dietitians, physical therapists, and other healthcare professionals to develop a comprehensive plan of care.

By assessing, documenting, and managing edema, nurses help patients achieve fluid balance, alleviate discomfort, and reduce the risk of complications. They play a critical role in providing patient education and support to promote self-management and prevent further accumulation of fluid in body tissues.

35. Electrocardiogram (EKG/ECG)

In nursing, an electrocardiogram (EKG or ECG) refers to a diagnostic test that measures the electrical activity of the heart. It is a non-invasive procedure that provides important information about the heart's function and can help identify various cardiac conditions or abnormalities.

During an electrocardiogram, electrodes are placed on specific areas of the patient's chest, arms, and legs to detect and record the electrical signals generated by the heart. The electrodes are connected to a machine that produces a graphical representation, known as an electrocardiogram, of the heart's electrical activity.

Nurses play a vital role in the electrocardiogram process, which includes the following responsibilities:

1. Preparation: Nurses prepare the patient for the procedure, ensuring that the skin is clean and dry where the electrodes will be placed. They explain the procedure, address any questions or concerns the patient may have, and ensure the patient is comfortable and properly positioned.

2. Electrode Placement: Nurses place the electrodes on the patient's chest, arms, and legs in specific locations as indicated by the healthcare provider. Correct placement is crucial for obtaining accurate readings. They may need to shave excess hair to ensure good electrode-skin contact and improve the quality of the recording.

3. Monitoring: Nurses monitor the patient throughout the electrocardiogram, ensuring that the electrodes remain in place and that the patient is comfortable. They observe for any signs of discomfort, allergies, or skin irritation related to the electrodes and address any concerns promptly.

4. Troubleshooting: If there are any technical difficulties during the recording, nurses troubleshoot the issue, ensuring that the machine is functioning properly and that the electrodes are securely attached.

5. Post-Procedure Care: Once the electrocardiogram is complete, nurses remove the electrodes and clean the patient's skin. They ensure that the results are documented accurately in the patient's medical record and communicate any pertinent findings to the healthcare team.

Nurses also collaborate with healthcare providers to analyze and interpret the electrocardiogram results. They may assist in identifying key patterns, abnormalities, or changes in the heart's electrical activity, which can provide valuable information for diagnosing and managing cardiac conditions.

Overall, nurses play a critical role in performing and assisting with electrocardiograms, ensuring patient safety, comfort, and accurate recording of the heart's electrical activity.

36. Electrolyte

In nursing, "electrolyte" refers to a chemical substance or mineral found in the body fluids, such as blood, urine, and cells, that carries an electric charge when dissolved in water. Electrolytes are essential for maintaining various bodily functions, including proper nerve and muscle function, maintaining fluid balance, and regulating pH levels.

The major electrolytes in the body include:

1. Sodium (Na+): Sodium plays a critical role in fluid balance, nerve function, and muscle contraction. It helps maintain normal blood pressure and regulates the amount of water in the body.

2. Potassium (K+): Potassium is crucial for nerve and muscle cell functioning, including regulating heart rhythm. It helps balance fluids, maintain optimal pH levels, and supports overall cellular function.

3. Calcium (Ca2+): Calcium is essential for strong bones and teeth, blood clotting, nerve function, and muscle contraction. It also plays a role in various enzymatic reactions and cell signaling.

4. Magnesium (Mg2+): Magnesium is involved in numerous biochemical reactions in the body, including energy production, nerve function, and muscle contraction. It also supports bone health and helps maintain a regular heart rhythm.

5. Chloride (Cl-): Chloride works with sodium and potassium to maintain proper fluid balance, regulate blood pressure, and support nerve function.

Nurses play a vital role in monitoring and managing electrolyte levels in patients. This includes:

1. Assessment: Nurses assess patients for signs and symptoms of electrolyte imbalances, such as muscle weakness, cardiac arrhythmias, changes in mental status, fatigue, dehydration, or abnormal lab results.

2. Monitoring and Lab Tests: Nurses closely monitor electrolyte levels through routine lab tests, such as blood tests or urine tests. They interpret the lab results, looking for abnormalities in electrolyte values, and report any significant deviations to the healthcare team.

3. Administration of Electrolyte Therapy: Depending on the specific electrolyte imbalance, nurses administer electrolyte replacement therapies, such as intravenous fluids, oral supplements, or medications, as prescribed by the healthcare provider.

4. Education: Nurses provide patient education on maintaining electrolyte balance through proper nutrition, fluid intake, and medication management. They may offer guidance on dietary sources of electrolytes and the importance of adhering to prescribed treatments or medications.

5. Collaboration: Nurses collaborate with the healthcare team, including physicians, dietitians, and pharmacists, to develop individualized care plans for managing electrolyte imbalances and promoting overall wellness.

By monitoring and managing electrolyte levels, nurses help maintain the body's proper functioning, prevent complications, and ensure patients receive appropriate treatments to restore electrolyte balance.

37. Embolism

Embolism in nursing refers to a medical condition in which an artery or a vein is blocked by a foreign substance, such as a blood clot, fat globule, air bubble, or a piece of tumor. It can result in the interruption of blood flow to a specific part of the body, leading to tissue damage or organ dysfunction. In nursing, understanding the signs, symptoms, and risk factors associated with embolism is crucial for prompt recognition, early intervention, and effective management of this potentially life-threatening condition. Nurses play a vital role in assessing patient risks, providing preventive measures, and administering appropriate care to minimize complications associated with embolism.

38. Endotracheal tube

Endotracheal tube (ET tube) in nursing refers to a flexible plastic tube that is inserted into the trachea through the mouth or nose to establish and maintain a patent airway and assist with artificial ventilation. It is used in cases where a patient requires mechanical ventilation due to respiratory failure, surgery, or other medical conditions. The ET tube is carefully inserted by trained healthcare professionals, such as nurses, to ensure proper placement and minimize complications. It is connected to a mechanical ventilator or a bag-valve-mask device to assist with the delivery of oxygen and removal of carbon dioxide from the patient's lungs. In nursing, understanding the indications, insertion techniques, monitoring, and care of patients with endotracheal tubes is essential for safe and effective respiratory management.

39. Epinephrine

Epinephrine, also known as adrenaline, is a medication commonly used in nursing to treat severe allergic reactions, anaphylaxis, asthma attacks, and cardiac arrest. It is a hormone and neurotransmitter that acts on various receptors in the body to increase heart rate, constrict blood vessels, dilate airways, and improve blood flow. In nursing, epinephrine is typically administered via injection or intravenous infusion, and its use requires careful monitoring of vital signs and potential side effects.

40. Erythema

In nursing, erythema is a term used to describe a skin condition characterized by redness or flushing. It occurs due to the dilation of blood vessels in the skin, which can be caused by various factors such as inflammation, allergic reactions, or increased blood flow. Erythema can occur as a standalone condition or as a symptom of an underlying disease or infection. In nursing, it is important to assess and document the presence and severity of erythema, as it may indicate an allergic reaction, infection, or an adverse reaction to medication. Nursing interventions for erythema may include applying topical creams or medications, providing comfort measures, and monitoring for any changes or worsening of the condition.

41. Fecal

In nursing, "fecal" refers to anything related to feces, which is the waste product expelled from the body through the rectum. Nurses may assess and monitor the characteristics of fecal matter, such as color, consistency, and odor, as it can provide information about a patient's gastrointestinal health. Nurses may also be responsible for assisting patients with managing and maintaining proper bowel movements, including monitoring stool frequency and performing interventions to promote regularity and prevent constipation or diarrhea.

42. Fever

In nursing, "fever" refers to a higher-than-normal body temperature. It is considered one of the vital signs that nurses monitor in patients. Typically, a fever is defined as a body temperature above 100.4°F (38°C) orally or above 99.5°F (37.5°C) rectally.

Nurses play a crucial role in assessing and managing fevers in patients. This includes monitoring the temperature regularly, identifying the underlying cause, and providing appropriate interventions to manage and reduce the fever. Nurses may administer antipyretic medications, such as acetaminophen or ibuprofen, to help lower the body temperature. They also assess for other signs and symptoms related to the fever, such as increased heart rate, dehydration, chills, or sweating, which can provide important information about the patient's condition. Nurses collaborate with other healthcare team members to develop a comprehensive care plan to address both the fever and its underlying cause.

43. Foley catheter

In nursing, a Foley catheter is a flexible tube that is inserted into the bladder to drain urine. It consists of a thin tube with an inflatable balloon at one end to hold it in place inside the bladder. The other end of the catheter is connected to a collection bag where urine can be collected and measured.

Nurses often use Foley catheters in a variety of clinical settings, such as in hospitals, nursing homes, and homecare, to assist patients who have difficulty urinating or who require accurate measurement of urine output. These may include patients who are bedridden, undergoing surgery, or experiencing conditions such as urinary retention or incontinence.

Nurses are responsible for the insertion and care of Foley catheters, ensuring proper technique and hygiene to minimize the risk of infection or injury. They regularly monitor and assess the catheter site, drainage, and urine output. Nurses also aim to maintain the patency of the catheter by regularly flushing it with sterile saline or water and ensuring the collection bag is positioned and emptied appropriately. When the Foley catheter is no longer needed, nurses are responsible for its removal while maintaining patient comfort and ensuring aseptic technique.

44. Fracture

In nursing, a fracture refers to a break or crack in a bone. Fractures can occur due to various reasons, such as falls, accidents, sports injuries, or underlying medical conditions like osteoporosis or cancer.

Nurses play a crucial role in the care of patients with fractures. This includes assessing and documenting the extent and location of the fracture, as well as monitoring for any associated symptoms such as pain, swelling, deformity, or impaired function. Nurses may also assess for any neurovascular compromise, such as numbness, tingling, weakness, or changes in pulse or color, which could indicate a more serious injury.

Nurses are involved in providing pain management interventions, such as administering pain medications and implementing non-pharmacological techniques like positioning and applying cold or heat therapy. They might assist with immobilization techniques like splints, casts, or traction, and monitor for any complications or adverse effects related to these interventions.

Additionally, nurses provide education to patients and their families on proper care and management of the fracture, such as the importance of mobility restrictions, weight-bearing limitations, and wound care. They also support the patient's physical and emotional recovery, provide assistance with activities of daily living, and may coordinate with other healthcare professionals, such as physical therapists or orthopedic specialists, to ensure comprehensive care for the patient with a fracture.

45. Gangrene

In nursing, gangrene is a condition characterized by the death and decay of body tissues due to a lack of blood supply or severe infection. It occurs when there is a disruption in the blood flow to a specific area, leading to tissue death and subsequential bacterial invasion. Gangrene can occur in various parts of the body, including the extremities, digestive system, or internal organs.

Nurses play a critical role in the management and care of patients with gangrene. This includes assessing and monitoring the affected area for signs and symptoms of gangrene, such as changes in skin color (e.g., black or purple), severe pain, foul-smelling discharge, or the presence of gas bubbles in the tissues.

Nurses assist with wound care by closely monitoring and documenting the progression of the gangrene, implementing appropriate interventions for wound management, and providing meticulous and frequent dressing changes. They work collaboratively with the healthcare team to administer antibiotics, provide analgesics for pain relief, and address any underlying conditions contributing to the development of gangrene.

Nurses also educate patients and their families on proper wound care, hygiene practices, and prevention strategies to minimize the risk of further complications. They play a vital role in promoting patient comfort and facilitating emotional support to patients dealing with the physical and psychological impact of gangrene. Additionally, nurses advocate for the prompt and appropriate interventions required to manage gangrene and prevent its spread, often coordinating with other healthcare professionals, such as wound care specialists or surgeons, to ensure comprehensive care for the patient.

46. Gastrointestinal

In nursing, "gastrointestinal" refers to the system in the body that is responsible for the digestion and absorption of food. It includes the organs and structures involved in this process, such as the mouth, esophagus, stomach, small intestine, large intestine (colon), rectum, and anus.

Nurses are involved in the assessment, management, and care of patients with gastrointestinal disorders or conditions. This includes monitoring and documenting symptoms related to the gastrointestinal system, such as abdominal pain, bloating, nausea, vomiting, diarrhea, constipation, or changes in bowel habits.

Nurses administer medications and treatments prescribed to manage gastrointestinal conditions, such as antacids for heartburn, antiemetics for nausea and vomiting, or laxatives for constipation. They also educate patients and their families on dietary modifications, including information on proper nutrition, hydration, and therapeutic diets that are tailored to specific gastrointestinal disorders or conditions.

Nurses support patients undergoing gastrointestinal procedures or surgeries, such as endoscopies, colonoscopies, or bowel resection, by providing pre-operative and post-operative care, monitoring vital signs, managing pain, and ensuring proper wound care.l

Furthermore, nurses play a vital role in promoting patient education and self-care management related to gastrointestinal health. This includes teaching patients about the importance of maintaining a healthy diet, regular exercise, and appropriate bowel habits to prevent gastrointestinal disorders. Nurses may also provide guidance on early detection and screening for conditions such as colorectal cancer.

47. Hematoma

In nursing, a hematoma refers to a localized collection of blood outside of blood vessels. It occurs when there is damage to blood vessels, leading to bleeding into the surrounding tissues. Hematomas can occur as a result of trauma, surgical procedures, bruises, or certain medical conditions.

Nurses play a role in the assessment and management of hematomas. This includes monitoring the affected area for signs and symptoms, such as swelling, discoloration (often appearing as a bruise), pain, or a firm lump under the skin. Nurses assess the size, shape, and consistency of the hematoma, as well as any signs of infection or complications.

In terms of management, nurses may employ interventions and treatments to promote healing and prevent further complications. Depending on the severity and location of the hematoma, this may include applying ice or heat therapy, elevating the affected area, providing pain relief medications, and using compression bandages or dressings.

Nurses also play a crucial role in education, providing patients and their families with information about the hematoma, its expected progression, and recommendations for self-care. They educate on the signs of complications or worsening symptoms that may require medical attention. Additionally, nurses collaborate with healthcare professionals, such as physicians or surgeons, to coordinate the appropriate management and follow-up care for patients with hematomas.

48. Hemorrhage

In nursing, a hemorrhage refers to excessive bleeding or the escape of blood from blood vessels, either internally or externally. Hemorrhages can occur due to trauma, surgical procedures, or underlying medical conditions, and they can vary in severity and location.

Nurses play a critical role in the assessment, prevention, and management of hemorrhages. This includes closely monitoring patients for signs and symptoms of bleeding, such as uncontrolled or excessive bleeding, decreased blood pressure, increased heart rate, pallor, dizziness, or altered mental status. Nurses also assess the patient's overall hemodynamic stability, including the presence of shock.

In terms of prevention, nurses take measures to minimize the risk of hemorrhage during procedures or interventions. This may involve confirming adequate blood clotting function, administering medications to promote clotting (such as clotting factors), and closely monitoring patients who are at a higher risk for hemorrhage due to certain medical conditions or medications.

In the event of a hemorrhage, nurses provide immediate interventions to control bleeding and stabilize the patient. This can include applying direct pressure to the site of bleeding, using compression dressings or tourniquets as appropriate, elevating the affected area, administering intravenous fluids or blood products, and coordinating with the healthcare team for emergent interventions, such as surgical procedures or interventions to stop the bleeding.

Nurses also play a crucial role in post-hemorrhage care, providing monitoring, wound care, and administering medications as prescribed. Additionally, they educate patients and their families on the signs of hemorrhage, including measures to prevent further bleeding or complications.

In severe cases or when complications arise, nurses collaborate with other healthcare professionals, such as surgeons or interventional radiologists, to provide comprehensive care and ongoing management for patients experiencing hemorrhage.

49. Hospice

In nursing, hospice refers to a specialized type of care provided to individuals who are facing a life-limiting illness, typically with a prognosis of six months or less to live. Hospice care focuses on providing comfort, support, and quality of life for patients in the final stages of their illness, as well as emotional and spiritual support for their families.

Hospice care can be provided in various settings, including patients' homes, nursing homes, or dedicated hospice facilities. The goal of hospice care is to manage symptoms, control pain, and ensure dignity and peace for patients during their remaining time. This often involves a multidisciplinary team approach, including nurses, doctors, social workers, chaplains, therapists, and other healthcare professionals, who work together to address the physical, emotional, and spiritual needs of the patient and their family.

Nurses in hospice care play an essential role in managing and coordinating the patient's care. They assess and monitor symptoms, provide pain management and symptom control medications, perform nursing interventions to enhance comfort (such as positioning and personal care), and offer emotional support to patients and their families. Nurses also work closely with the patient's family to educate them about the dying process, assist with making end-of-life decisions, and provide guidance on bereavement support.

Furthermore, nurses in hospice care act as advocates and liaisons for patients, communicating with other healthcare professionals and ensuring that the patient's wishes and goals of care are respected and honored. They collaborate with the interdisciplinary hospice team to develop an individualized care plan and ensure continuity of care.

Overall, hospice care provided by nurses is focused on enhancing quality of life for patients in their final stages of illness and providing compassionate support that addresses the physical, emotional, and spiritual needs of both the patient and their loved ones.

50. Hypertension

Hypotension in nursing refers to low blood pressure, which is a condition characterized by a decrease in the force of blood being pumped by the heart against the blood vessel walls. In nursing, hypotension is a vital sign that nurses regularly monitor and assess. There are various causes of hypotension, including dehydration, medication side effects, heart problems, hormonal imbalances, and excessive bleeding. In some cases, hypotension can be a symptom of an underlying medical condition or a potentially life-threatening emergency.

Nurses play a significant role in identifying and managing hypotension. They assess blood pressure readings and monitor patients for symptoms of low blood pressure, such as dizziness, lightheadedness, fainting, confusion, and rapid heartbeat. Nurses may collaborate with healthcare providers to determine the underlying cause of hypotension and develop a care plan to address it. The interventions may include administering intravenous fluids, adjusting medications, optimizing hydration, and maintaining a safe environment to prevent falls or injuries associated with low blood pressure.

51. Hypotension

In nursing, hypotension refers to a lower-than-normal blood pressure reading. Blood pressure is the force exerted by blood against the walls of blood vessels, and it is an essential vital sign that helps evaluate a person's cardiovascular health.

Hypotension is typically defined as a systolic blood pressure (the top number) below 90 mmHg or a diastolic blood pressure (the bottom number) below 60 mmHg. However, the specific values used to define hypotension may vary depending on the individual and the clinical context.

Nurses play a crucial role in assessing, monitoring, and managing patients with hypotension. This includes regularly measuring a patient's blood pressure using appropriate techniques and equipment. Nurses also observe for signs and symptoms associated with hypotension, such as dizziness, lightheadedness, fatigue, confusion, blurred vision, or fainting.

In terms of management, nurses work to identify the underlying cause of hypotension and implement appropriate interventions. These interventions may vary depending on the severity and cause of the low blood pressure but can include measures such as repositioning the patient, administering fluids via intravenous infusion, adjusting medications, or using vasopressor medications to increase blood pressure.

Nurses also provide education to patients and their families about hypotension, including information about lifestyle modifications, medication management, and the importance of seeking medical attention if symptoms worsen or new symptoms develop. They may also collaborate with other healthcare professionals, such as physicians or pharmacists, to optimize the care and management of patients with hypotension.

52. Hypoxia

In nursing, hypoxia refers to a condition in which there is an inadequate supply of oxygen to the body's tissues and cells. It occurs when there is a decrease in the amount of oxygen reaching the organs and tissues or when there is impaired oxygen utilization at the cellular level.

Nurses play a crucial role in recognizing and managing hypoxia. They assess patients for signs and symptoms associated with hypoxia, such as shortness of breath, rapid breathing, cyanosis (blue tint to the skin), confusion, restlessness, fatigue, or changes in vital signs.

When hypoxia is suspected, nurses intervene by providing supplemental oxygen therapy to increase the oxygen concentration in the patient's inspired air. This may involve administering oxygen through nasal cannulas, masks, or other specialized devices, depending on the patient's condition and needs.

Nurses also assess and monitor the patient's respiratory status, oxygen saturation levels (using pulse oximetry), and other vital signs. They collaborate with other healthcare professionals to identify the underlying cause of hypoxia, such as respiratory conditions, cardiac dysfunction, anemia, or circulatory problems, and implement appropriate treatments or interventions.

In addition to providing immediate interventions, nurses educate patients and their families about hypoxia, its causes, and preventive measures. They provide guidance on breathing exercises, positioning techniques, smoking cessation, and lifestyle modifications to optimize oxygenation and prevent further episodes of hypoxia.

Nurses also advocate for patients by ensuring timely and appropriate interventions to address and manage hypoxia. They collaborate with the healthcare team to monitor the patient's response to interventions, adjust the oxygen therapy as needed, and address any potential complications or side effects associated with oxygen administration.

53. Incision

In nursing, an incision refers to a deliberate cut made into the skin and underlying tissues during a surgical procedure. Incisions are made to access and treat underlying structures or organs, remove a growth or tumor, repair damaged tissues, or perform other necessary procedures.

Nurses play a role in the care of patients who have undergone surgical incisions. This includes assessing and monitoring the incision site for signs of infection or complications, such as redness, swelling, drainage, or increased pain. Nurses also monitor vital signs, including temperature, which can indicate the presence of infection.

Nurses are responsible for providing appropriate wound care for the incision. This may involve dressing changes, cleaning the incision site, and applying sterile techniques to prevent infection. Nurses also educate patients and their families on incision care, including instructions for keeping the incision clean and dry, recognizing signs of infection, and understanding any activity restrictions or precautions related to the surgical incision.

In addition to incision care, nurses provide pain management interventions to ensure patient comfort. This may involve administering prescribed pain medications, implementing non-pharmacological pain relief measures, and assisting patients with positioning or movement techniques that minimize discomfort.

Nurses collaborate with the healthcare team, including surgeons and other providers, to ensure proper management and healing of the incision. They communicate any concerns or changes in the incision's appearance or symptoms to the appropriate healthcare professionals.

Overall, nurses play an important role in monitoring, managing, and educating patients about incisions to promote proper healing, prevent complications, and support patients' overall recovery after surgery.

54. Infection

In nursing, infection refers to the invasion and multiplication of microorganisms, such as bacteria, viruses, fungi, or parasites, in a host's body. Infections can occur in various areas of the body, both externally and internally, and can lead to localized or systemic symptoms and complications.

Nurses play a crucial role in identifying, preventing, and managing infections in healthcare settings. They are responsible for assessing patients for signs and symptoms of infection, such as fever, chills, redness, swelling, pain, drainage, or changes in vital signs. Nurses also take into account the patient's medical history, risk factors, and recent procedures or exposures to determine the likelihood of infection.

When an infection is suspected or confirmed, nurses implement appropriate infection prevention and control measures. This includes adhering to proper hand hygiene protocols, using personal protective equipment (such as gloves, masks, and gowns) when necessary, and following established isolation precautions to prevent the spread of infection.

Nurses also assist with infection management by administering prescribed antibiotics or antiviral medications, monitoring the patient's response to treatment, and providing wound care or other interventions to promote healing and prevent further infection. They may collect specimens for laboratory testing to identify the causative microorganism of the infection.

In addition to direct patient care, nurses educate patients and their families about infection prevention strategies and the importance of adhering to prescribed medications and treatments. Nurses also play a role in advocating for appropriate infection control practices within their healthcare settings, including educating other healthcare professionals on best practices and participating in quality improvement initiatives to reduce the risk of healthcare-associated infections.

Overall, nurses in infection control play a critical role in the identification, prevention, and management of infections. They work collaboratively with the healthcare team to minimize the spread of infection, provide evidence-based care to infected individuals, and educate patients and their families on infection prevention strategies.

55. Inflammation

In nursing, inflammation refers to the body's natural response to injury, infection, or irritation. It is a complex biological process that involves the activation of the immune system and the release of various chemical mediators.

Nurses play a vital role in recognizing, assessing, and managing inflammation in patients. They assess patients for signs and symptoms of inflammation, such as redness, swelling, heat, pain, and loss of function in the affected area. Nurses also monitor vital signs, laboratory values, and changes in overall health status that may indicate an inflammatory response.

When inflammation is present, nurses intervene by providing treatments aimed at reducing or managing inflammation. This may include administering anti-inflammatory medications, applying cold or heat therapy, providing wound care, or assisting with pain management techniques.

Nurses also educate patients and their families about inflammation and its management. This includes explaining the benefits and potential side effects of prescribed medications, teaching proper wound care techniques, and providing guidance on lifestyle modifications that can help reduce inflammation, such as maintaining a healthy diet, regular exercise, and stress management.

In cases of chronic inflammation, nurses may work closely with other healthcare professionals, such as physicians or specialists, to develop a comprehensive care plan. This may involve coordinating medications, therapies, and rehabilitation services to manage the underlying condition contributing to chronic inflammation and improve overall patient outcomes.

Additionally, nurses advocate for and support patients in managing inflammation by promoting adherence to prescribed treatments, providing education on the importance of following healthcare providers' recommendations, and addressing any concerns or questions patients may have.

Overall, nurses in inflammation management play an essential role in assessing, managing, and educating patients about inflammation. They work collaboratively with the healthcare team to provide evidence-based care that helps reduce inflammation, alleviate symptoms, and support patients in their journey to recovery.

56. Infusion

In nursing, infusion refers to the administration of fluids, medications, or other substances directly into a patient's bloodstream using intravenous (IV) techniques. Infusion therapy is commonly used in a variety of healthcare settings to provide rapid and controlled delivery of fluids and medications when oral administration is not feasible or effective.

Nurses play a critical role in administering infusions and ensuring patient safety throughout the process. This includes assessing the patient's fluid and medication needs, selecting the appropriate infusion device and equipment, and preparing and administering the infusion according to established protocols and guidelines.

Nurses monitor the patient's vital signs, including blood pressure, heart rate, and oxygen saturation, to assess the response to the infusion and ensure that the patient is tolerating it well. They also observe for signs of adverse reactions, such as allergic reactions or fluid overload, and respond promptly if any issues arise.

In addition, nurses closely monitor the infusion site, assessing for signs of complications or infections, and ensure that the infusion is running at the prescribed rate. They often perform dressing changes and site care to maintain the integrity of the IV site and prevent infection.

Nurses also educate patients and their families about the purpose and management of the infusion. This includes providing information about the infusion therapy, potential side effects, signs and symptoms to monitor for, and self-care techniques related to the infusion site.

Nurses collaborate with other healthcare professionals, such as pharmacists and physicians, to ensure that the infusion therapy is appropriate for the patient's condition and individual needs. They communicate any changes or concerns related to the infusion therapy and work as advocates to ensure that patients receive safe and effective care.

Overall, infusion in nursing involves the safe administration and monitoring of fluids and medications through the IV route. Nurses play a crucial role in the assessment, management, and education related to infusion therapy to promote patient safety and optimize treatment outcomes.

57. Inpatient

In nursing, an inpatient refers to a person who has been admitted to a hospital or healthcare facility for medical or surgical treatment and requires care and monitoring on an ongoing basis. In contrast, an outpatient refers to a person who visits a healthcare facility for medical services but does not require admission or an overnight stay.

Nurses in an inpatient setting are responsible for providing comprehensive care to patients during their hospital stay. This includes assessing, planning, implementing, and evaluating nursing interventions to address the patient's needs and promote their recovery.

Nurses in an inpatient setting collaborate with the interdisciplinary healthcare team, including physicians, specialists, pharmacists, and other healthcare professionals, to develop and implement a holistic care plan for each patient. They monitor the patient's condition, vital signs, and response to treatments or medications. Nurses administer medications, provide wound care, assist with activities of daily living, and provide emotional support to patients and their families.

In addition to direct patient care, nurses in an inpatient setting also play a role in patient education. They provide information regarding the patient's diagnosis, treatments, and self-care management during and after their hospital stay. They also educate patients and families about discharge instructions, medications, follow-up appointments, and any necessary lifestyle modifications.

Furthermore, nurses in an inpatient setting coordinate and facilitate communication among the healthcare team, ensure that documentation is complete and accurate, and advocate for patients' rights and needs. They prioritize patient safety, infection control, and quality of care.

Overall, nurses in an inpatient setting provide continuous care, support, and education to patients who require hospitalization for medical or surgical interventions. They collaborate with the healthcare team to ensure that patients receive optimal care and achieve the best possible outcomes during their inpatient stay.

58. IV (intravenous)

In nursing, IV (intravenous) refers to the administration of fluids, medications, or other substances directly into a patient's vein using a needle or catheter. It is a common method of delivering fast and efficient treatment when oral administration is not feasible, or when immediate effects are required.

The process of administering IV involves inserting an IV catheter into a patient's vein, typically in the hand, arm, or other suitable site. The catheter is connected to a sterile IV tubing, which is then attached to a bag or container of fluids or medications.

Nurses play a crucial role in IV therapy. They assess the patient's vital signs, medical history, and the prescribed treatment to determine the appropriate type and rate of IV fluid and medication administration. Nurses ensure that the solutions used are compatible with the patient's condition and monitor the patient's response to the IV therapy.

Nurses also monitor the IV site for signs of complications, such as infection, infiltration (leakage into surrounding tissues), or phlebitis (inflammation of the vein). They regularly check the infusion site, assess for any redness, swelling, pain, or other signs of complications, and take appropriate actions, such as adjusting the catheter or initiating site care, as needed.

Additionally, nurses are responsible for ensuring that the IV infusion is running at the prescribed rate and that the solutions and medications are properly labeled and prepared. They assess the patient's tolerance to the IV therapy, monitor for any adverse reactions or side effects, and promptly address any concerns or complications that may arise.

Nurses also educate patients and their families about the purpose of the IV therapy, its potential side effects, and how to care for the IV site during and after the infusion period. Patients are often taught to recognize signs of infection or other complications, as well as to understand the importance of maintaining the integrity of the IV site.

In summary, IV (intravenous) therapy in nursing involves the administration of fluids, medications, or other substances directly into a patient's vein. Nurses oversee the entire process, including assessing the patient, selecting and preparing the appropriate IV solutions and medications, monitoring the infusion, and providing patient education and care to ensure safe and effective IV therapy.

59. Isolation

In nursing, isolation refers to the practice of implementing specific precautions and measures to prevent the spread of infectious diseases or to protect vulnerable patients from acquiring infections. Isolation protocols are designed to minimize the transmission of pathogens in healthcare settings and to ensure the safety of both patients and healthcare providers.

Isolation precautions are categorized into different types, including standard precautions, transmission-based precautions, and additional precautions specific to certain infectious diseases. These precautions involve various measures, such as hand hygiene, wearing personal protective equipment (e.g., gloves, masks, gowns), practicing respiratory etiquette (e.g., covering mouth and nose when coughing or sneezing), and implementing appropriate disinfection and sterilization procedures.

Nurses play a critical role in implementing and maintaining isolation measures. They assess and identify patients who require isolation precautions based on their medical condition, symptoms, or the type of infectious agent involved. Nurses ensure that patients are placed in suitable isolation rooms or areas that provide the necessary infection control measures, such as adequate ventilation or negative pressure rooms for airborne infections.

Nurses adhere to the recommended isolation precautions and educate patients, families, and visitors on the importance of following these measures to prevent the transmission of pathogens. They communicate with the healthcare team, including physicians, infection prevention specialists, and environmental services, to ensure that proper protocols are followed and that any additional measures are implemented when necessary.

In addition, nurses provide emotional support and care to patients in isolation, as the experience can be isolating, stressful, and anxiety-inducing. Nurses may use effective communication techniques and therapeutic interventions to lessen patients' fears and address their psychosocial needs during isolation.

Nurses are also responsible for educating and training healthcare providers on proper isolation techniques and infection control practices. They actively contribute to ongoing infection control initiatives and quality improvement efforts within the healthcare facility.

Overall, nurses are integral to the implementation and maintenance of isolation precautions. They work collaboratively with the healthcare team to ensure that appropriate measures are in place to prevent the spread of infectious diseases and to promote the well-being and safety of all patients and healthcare providers.

60. Jaundice

Jaundice is a condition characterized by the yellowing of the skin and eyes due to high levels of bilirubin in the bloodstream. It occurs when there is a disruption in the normal processing of bilirubin by the liver, leading to its accumulation in the body. In nursing, jaundice is an important condition to monitor and manage as it can be a sign of various underlying liver diseases or other medical conditions. Nurses play a critical role in assessing the severity of jaundice, monitoring liver function tests, providing appropriate medical interventions, and educating patients and their families about the condition and its management.

61. Joint

In nursing, a joint refers to the area where two or more bones meet and are connected to each other. Joints allow for movement and flexibility in the body. Nurses often assess and monitor the condition of joints, especially in patients with musculoskeletal disorders, injuries, or chronic conditions such as arthritis. They may check for signs of inflammation, pain, stiffness, or limited range of motion in the joints. Nurses may also assist patients with joint exercises or recommend interventions to manage or alleviate joint pain, such as hot or cold therapy, medication, or physical therapy.

62. Laceration

In nursing, a laceration refers to a type of wound characterized by a tear or separation in the skin, typically caused by a sharp object or trauma. Lacerations can vary in severity, from small and superficial cuts to deep and extensive injuries that may involve underlying tissues, muscles, or organs.

Nurses play a crucial role in the assessment, management, and care of lacerations. This includes evaluating the size, depth, and location of the laceration, assessing for any associated damage or bleeding, and determining the need for further medical intervention such as stitches or sutures. Nurses also help to clean and dress the laceration, provide pain management, and educate patients on wound care and signs of infection. In some cases, they may also assist with procedures such as wound irrigation or wound closure. Additionally, nurses often provide education on wound healing, scar prevention, and follow-up care to promote optimal recovery.

63. Larynx

In nursing, the larynx refers to the part of the respiratory system commonly known as the voice box. It is located in the throat and plays a crucial role in voice production, as well as protecting the airway during swallowing and preventing food or liquid from entering the lungs.

Nurses may encounter patients with various conditions or issues related to the larynx. For instance, they may assess and manage patients with laryngitis (inflammation of the larynx), vocal cord nodules or polyps, laryngeal cancer, or injuries to the larynx. Nurses may assist in procedures such as laryngoscopy to visualize the larynx and assess its condition. They can also provide support and education to patients regarding voice rest, hydration, proper vocal technique, and lifestyle modifications to promote laryngeal health. Additionally, nurses may work collaboratively with speech therapists or otolaryngologists in the management and care of patients with laryngeal conditions.

Please note that while I strive to provide accurate information, it is always recommended to consult with a healthcare professional or refer to your nursing textbooks or resources for precise definitions and information.

64. Lavage

Lavage in nursing refers to a medical procedure that involves the flushing or irrigation of a body cavity or hollow organ with fluid. This is typically done to clean the area, remove debris or toxins, collect samples for analysis, or administer medication directly to the site. Lavage can be performed on various body parts such as the stomach, bladder, lungs, sinuses, or wounds, and it is often used in the management of certain medical conditions or during surgical procedures.

65. Lesion

In nursing, a lesion refers to a specific area of abnormal tissue on or within the body. It can be a change in the skin, mucous membranes, or internal organs that is different from the surrounding healthy tissue. Lesions can have various causes, including infections, traumas, tumors, autoimmune diseases, or other pathological processes.

Nurses use the term lesion to describe and document the size, location, appearance, and characteristics of these abnormal tissue areas. They assess and monitor lesions for changes in size, shape, color, texture, or other features that may indicate improvement or deterioration of the underlying condition. Nurses may also perform interventions to manage lesions, such as wound care, administration of topical or systemic medications, or coordination with other healthcare professionals for further evaluation or treatment.

66. Ligament

In nursing, a ligament refers to a connective tissue structure that connects bone to bone, providing stability and support to joints. Ligaments are made up of dense fibrous tissue and play a crucial role in maintaining the integrity and proper function of the musculoskeletal system.

Nurses may encounter ligament injuries in various clinical settings, such as sports medicine, orthopedics, or emergency departments. Common examples of ligament injuries include sprains, strains, or tears that occur due to trauma, overuse, or repetitive stress on a joint. Nurses may assess and monitor these injuries for signs of swelling, pain, limited range of motion, or instability. They may also educate patients about proper care and management of ligament injuries, which can involve rest, ice, compression, elevation (RICE), immobilization, physical therapy, or, in severe cases, surgical intervention.

Understanding ligament anatomy and function is important for nurses to provide appropriate care and support to patients with ligament injuries or conditions.

67. Lungs

In nursing, "lungs" refers to the pair of organs responsible for respiration, located in the chest. Nurses often assess and monitor the function of the lungs as part of their routine care, which may include listening for breath sounds, assessing oxygen levels, and monitoring respiratory rate. Evaluating the condition of the lungs helps nurses and healthcare professionals identify any abnormalities or respiratory issues and provide appropriate care.

68. Malnutrition

In nursing, "malnutrition" refers to a condition where a person's body does not receive adequate nutrition to support proper health and functioning. Malnutrition occurs when a person's diet lacks essential nutrients such as proteins, carbohydrates, fats, vitamins, and minerals. This can result from various factors including insufficient food intake, a diet lacking in nutrient-rich foods, or underlying medical conditions that affect nutrient absorption or metabolism.

Nurses play a crucial role in identifying and managing malnutrition in their patients. They assess patients' nutritional status, monitor weight changes, perform dietary evaluations, and collaborate with other healthcare professionals to develop appropriate nutrition plans. Nurses often provide education and counseling to patients and their caregivers regarding essential nutrients, dietary requirements, meal planning, and ways to improve nutritional intake. They also monitor the response to nutritional interventions and make necessary adjustments to optimize the patient's overall health and well-being.

69. Malignant

In nursing, "malignant" refers to a characteristic or quality of a disease or condition that is indicative of cancer or a cancerous growth. Malignant tumors or cells have the potential to invade nearby tissues or spread to other parts of the body, leading to the development and progression of cancer.

Nurses play a vital role in the care and management of patients with malignant conditions. They assist in the diagnosis and staging of cancers by collecting relevant health histories, conducting physical assessments, and carrying out various diagnostic tests. Nurses also provide education and support to patients and their families, explaining treatment options, potential side effects, and the overall prognosis.

Throughout the cancer journey, nurses provide symptom management, administer treatments such as chemotherapy or radiation therapy, monitor for complications or adverse reactions, and offer emotional support to patients and their loved ones. Additionally, they collaborate with other healthcare professionals to ensure comprehensive, holistic care for individuals affected by malignant conditions.

70. Metastasis

In nursing, "metastasis" refers to the spread of cancer from its original site to other parts of the body. When cancerous cells break away from the primary tumor, they can travel through the bloodstream or lymphatic system and form new tumors in distant organs or tissues. This process is known as metastasis.

Nurses play a crucial role in managing patients with metastatic cancer. They assist in monitoring and assessing patients for signs and symptoms of metastasis, such as the development of new tumors, pain, organ dysfunction, or other systemic effects. Nurses may collaborate with other healthcare professionals to perform diagnostic tests, imaging studies, or biopsies to confirm the presence and extent of metastatic disease.

Nurses also provide supportive care to patients with metastatic cancer, including symptom management, pain management, and emotional support. They educate patients and caregivers about the disease progression, treatment options, and potential side effects. Nurses often work closely with oncologists, surgeons, and other specialists to coordinate and implement a comprehensive treatment plan that focuses on managing symptoms, optimizing quality of life, and addressing the unique needs and goals of each patient.

71. Mucus

In nursing, "mucus" refers to a sticky substance that is produced by the mucous membranes lining various parts of the body, including the respiratory tract, digestive tract, and reproductive tract. Mucus serves several important functions, such as protecting and lubricating these tissues, trapping and removing foreign particles, and moisturizing and humidifying the surrounding environment.

In the context of nursing, mucus is often assessed in patients when evaluating their respiratory health. Nurses may observe and assess the quantity, color, consistency, and odor of mucus or sputum during physical examinations, especially when patients exhibit coughing, congestion, or other respiratory symptoms. These assessments can provide valuable information about the presence of infections, inflammation, or other respiratory conditions.

Nurses may assist patients with techniques to manage or clear mucus, such as deep breathing exercises, coughing techniques, or controlled coughing. They may also provide education and guidance on ways to maintain respiratory hygiene and prevent the accumulation of excess mucus. Monitoring changes in mucus production or characteristics can help nurses identify changes in a patient's condition and inform appropriate interventions or treatments.

72. Myocardial infarction (MI)

In nursing, "myocardial infarction (MI)" refers to a medical term commonly known as a heart attack. It occurs when there is a blockage of blood flow to a part of the heart muscle, leading to the death of heart tissue due to insufficient oxygen supply.

Nurses play a crucial role in the care of patients with myocardial infarction. They are often involved in the early recognition and assessment of symptoms, such as chest pain, shortness of breath, sweating, and discomfort in the upper body, as well as in monitoring vital signs and performing electrocardiograms (ECGs or EKGs). Nurses also administer medications as prescribed to relieve pain, restore blood flow, and prevent further complications.

Additionally, nurses provide education to patients and their families about risk factors, lifestyle modifications, medications, and post-heart attack care. They assist in the management of associated conditions like hypertension, diabetes, and hyperlipidemia, as well as provide emotional support and counseling during the recovery process. Nurses help monitor and promote cardiac rehabilitation and guide patients in adopting healthy habits to reduce the risk of future myocardial infarctions or heart-related complications.

73. Nasogastric tube

In nursing, a "nasogastric tube" refers to a medical device that is inserted through the nose and down into the stomach. It is commonly used for various purposes, such as providing nutrition, hydration, or medication, decompressing the stomach, or removing fluids or toxins from the gastrointestinal tract.

Nurses often play a significant role in the management of patients with nasogastric tubes. They assess the appropriateness and need for the tube, ensure proper insertion technique, and monitor the patient's tolerance and response to the tube. Nurses also verify the correct placement of the tube by assessing pH levels or conducting an X-ray, as misplacement could result in complications.

Nurses provide ongoing care for patients with nasogastric tubes, including monitoring tube position and patency, administering prescribed fluids or medications, and checking for signs of complications such as tube dislodgement, blockage, or aspiration. They are responsible for maintaining proper hygiene and securing the tube in place to prevent accidental removal or displacement. Nurses may provide education to patients and their families about the purpose, care, and potential risks associated with the nasogastric tube.

Furthermore, nurses collaborate with other healthcare professionals to assess the patient's nutritional needs, calculate appropriate feeding regimens, and adjust the tube feedings as necessary. They also ensure that patients receive proper education and training on the use and maintenance of the nasogastric tube if it is intended for home or continued care.

74. Nausea

In nursing, "nausea" refers to a sensation of discomfort or unease in the stomach, often associated with an involuntary urge to vomit. Nausea can be caused by various factors, including illness, medication side effects, emotional distress, or physiological changes.

Nurses frequently encounter patients experiencing nausea and play an essential role in assessing and managing this symptom. They assess the severity and duration of nausea, associated factors, and any potential complications. Nurses may use standardized assessment tools to measure and document the intensity of nausea to guide treatment interventions.

In treating nausea, nurses may suggest simple interventions such as deep breathing, distractions, or changes in position to help alleviate symptoms. They can also administer prescribed medications like antiemetics (anti-nausea drugs) to provide relief, such as ondansetron or promethazine. Additionally, nurses closely monitor patients for any signs of dehydration or worsening symptoms.

Nurses also provide patient education on strategies to manage nausea, including dietary modifications (such as eating smaller, more frequent meals), avoiding triggers, practicing stress-reducing techniques, and adhering to prescribed medication regimens. By addressing the patient's individual needs and employing evidence-based interventions, nurses aim to effectively manage and minimize the discomfort associated with nausea.

75. Nebulizer

In nursing, a "nebulizer" refers to a medical device used to deliver medication in the form of a mist or aerosol to the lungs. It is commonly used to treat respiratory conditions, such as asthma, chronic obstructive pulmonary disease (COPD), or other bronchial or lung disorders.

Nurses frequently use nebulizers in various care settings, including hospitals, clinics, and home care. They play a vital role in administering medication via a nebulizer and monitoring the patient's response to the treatment.

The nebulizer works by converting liquid medication into a fine mist that can be inhaled through a mask or mouthpiece. Nurses are responsible for setting up and preparing the nebulizer device, ensuring that it is functioning correctly, and verifying the proper medication and dosage.

Nurses also educate patients and their families on the correct use of the nebulizer, including demonstrating how to use and clean the equipment properly. They explain the purpose and expected benefits of the nebulizer treatment, potential side effects, and precautions. Additionally, nurses may assess the patient's lung function, monitor vital signs, and document the effectiveness of the nebulizer treatment.

Nurses collaborate with other healthcare professionals to ensure that patients receive appropriate medication prescriptions and develop individualized care plans. They continuously evaluate the patient's respiratory status and adjust the nebulizer treatment as necessary to optimize respiratory function and improve overall patient well-being.

76. NPO (nothing by mouth)

In nursing, "NPO" stands for "nothing by mouth." It is a medical order that instructs the patient not to consume any food or liquids orally for a specific period. The NPO status may be temporary or permanent, depending on the patient's condition or the purpose of the restriction.

Nurses play a key role in implementing and monitoring the NPO status as per the healthcare provider's orders. They ensure that patients understand and adhere to the NPO instructions, often providing education and support to minimize discomfort or anxiety.

During the NPO period, nurses monitor the patient's hydration status and administer intravenous fluids if necessary. They closely observe for any signs of dehydration, such as dry mouth, decreased urine output, or changes in vital signs. Nurses also assess the patient's nutritional needs and collaborate with dietitians or healthcare providers to develop alternative feeding plans, such as nasogastric tube feedings or parenteral nutrition, if appropriate.

Nurses carefully document the NPO status, including the start and end times, as well as any exceptions or modifications to the restriction. They communicate and collaborate with other healthcare team members to ensure the patient's safety and comfort during the NPO period. Additionally, nurses closely monitor patients' responses to the NPO status and promptly report any concerns or complications to the healthcare provider for further assessment and intervention.

77. Nutrients

In nursing, "nutrients" refer to substances found in food that are essential for the body's growth, development, maintenance, and overall function. Nutrients provide the necessary energy and raw materials for cellular processes, support bodily functions, and help maintain optimal health.

Nurses play a crucial role in understanding and educating patients about the importance of nutrients in maintaining overall well-being. They assess patients' nutritional status, including factors such as dietary intake, weight, body composition, and laboratory values. Nurses also collaborate with dietitians or other healthcare professionals to develop personalized nutrition plans or interventions based on individual needs and medical conditions.

Understanding the different types of nutrients is essential in nursing practice. There are macronutrients, including carbohydrates, proteins, and fats, which provide energy and serve various cellular functions. Micronutrients, such as vitamins and minerals, are required in smaller quantities for specific bodily functions, such as metabolism, immune function, and tissue repair.

Nurses educate patients about the importance of a balanced diet that includes all essential nutrients and may offer guidance on specific dietary modifications based on patient needs. They provide information about nutrient-rich food sources and appropriate portion sizes, helping patients make informed choices to meet their nutritional requirements.

Monitoring and evaluating the patient's response to nutritional interventions are also essential nursing responsibilities. Nurses assess for signs of malnutrition, monitor weight changes, evaluate laboratory values, and provide ongoing support or adjustments to the nutrition plan.

Overall, nurses understand the significant role nutrients play in promoting and maintaining good health and work collaboratively with other healthcare professionals to ensure patients receive adequate nutrition to support their overall well-being.

78. Oncology

Oncology in nursing refers to the specialized field of nursing focused on caring for patients diagnosed with cancer. Oncology nurses play a crucial role in the multidisciplinary care of patients throughout their cancer journey, including prevention, diagnosis, treatment, and survivorship or end-of-life care.

Oncology nurses possess specialized knowledge and skills to provide comprehensive care to patients with various types of cancer. They work closely with oncologists, surgeons, radiologists, and other healthcare professionals to ensure the best possible outcomes for their patients.

In the field of oncology nursing, nurses perform a range of responsibilities, including:

1. Patient assessment: Oncology nurses assess patients' physical, emotional, and psychological health to develop individualized care plans.

2. Treatment administration: They administer chemotherapy, radiation therapy, targeted therapies, immunotherapies, and other cancer treatments as prescribed by

physicians. Nurses also monitor patients' response to treatment and manage any side effects.

3. Symptom management: Oncology nurses help manage cancer-related symptoms such as pain, nausea, fatigue, and other treatment-related side effects.

4. Patient education and support: They provide education to patients and their families about the disease, treatment options, self-care, and community resources. Oncology nurses also offer emotional support and counseling, addressing the psychosocial needs of patients and their families.

5. Coordination of care: Oncology nurses collaborate with other healthcare professionals to coordinate various aspects of patient care, including scheduling appointments, coordinating tests, and ensuring effective communication among the healthcare team.

Oncology nursing requires a compassionate and empathetic approach, as nurses often support patients and their families through challenging physical and emotional experiences throughout the cancer journey. Continuous learning and staying up-to-date with advancements in cancer treatment and care are essential for oncology nurses to provide the highest standard of patient care.

79. Ophthalmoscope

An ophthalmoscope is a specialized medical instrument used by healthcare professionals, including nurses, to examine the interior structures of the eye. It allows for direct visualization of the retina, optic nerve, blood vessels, and other structures within the eye.

In the field of nursing, ophthalmoscopes are often utilized by nurses who work in ophthalmology or primary care settings. Here's how an ophthalmoscope is used in nursing:

1. Eye examinations: Nurses may use an ophthalmoscope during routine eye examinations to assess the health of the eyes. This can include checking for abnormalities, damage, or signs of conditions such as glaucoma, diabetic retinopathy, or macular degeneration.

2. Assessing visual abnormalities: Nurses may also use an ophthalmoscope to evaluate visual abnormalities, such as changes in the optic nerve or retina. This can help in diagnosing and managing conditions that affect vision.

3. Monitoring eye diseases: Ophthalmoscopes are often used to monitor the progression of eye diseases or conditions. Nurses can track changes in the retina or optic nerve over time, providing valuable information for treatment planning and management.

4. Documenting findings: Nurses use ophthalmoscopes to document their findings during eye examinations. This includes recording any abnormalities or changes in the eye structures, which helps in maintaining thorough and accurate patient records.

It's important for nurses using an ophthalmoscope to have a good understanding of the normal anatomy of the eye and how to properly use the instrument. Regular training and practice are necessary to ensure accurate assessment and interpretation of findings.

Additionally, nurses should follow infection control protocols by properly cleaning and disinfecting the ophthalmoscope between patients to prevent the spread of infections.

80. Orthopedic

Orthopedic nursing is a specialized field of nursing that focuses on the care of patients with musculoskeletal conditions, disorders, injuries, or surgeries. Orthopedic nurses provide comprehensive care to patients across the lifespan, ranging from infants with congenital orthopedic conditions to older adults with age-related musculoskeletal issues.

In the field of nursing, orthopedic nurses play a vital role in providing holistic care throughout the orthopedic care continuum, which includes preoperative, intraoperative, and postoperative phases. Here's what orthopedic nursing entails:

1. Preoperative care: Orthopedic nurses assess patients' medical history, perform physical examinations, and collaborate with the surgical team to develop a plan of care. This involves educating patients about the upcoming procedure, addressing their concerns, and preparing them mentally and physically for surgery.

2. Intraoperative care: Orthopedic nurses may assist the surgical team in the operating room during orthopedic procedures. They help maintain a sterile environment, ensure patient safety, and provide necessary supplies and instruments to the surgical team.

3. Postoperative care: After surgery, orthopedic nurses closely monitor patients' vital signs, surgical incisions, pain levels, and overall recovery progress. They administer medications, manage pain, provide wound care, and assist with early mobilization and rehabilitation. Orthopedic nurses also educate patients and their families on postoperative care instructions, as well as potential complications to watch for.

4. Musculoskeletal assessments: Orthopedic nurses conduct thorough assessments of musculoskeletal function. They evaluate joint mobility, muscle strength, sensation, and overall skeletal alignment to identify any abnormalities, injuries, or changes in condition. These assessments help in formulating individualized care plans and interventions.

5. Patient and family education: Orthopedic nurses play a crucial role in educating patients and their families about the diagnosis, treatment options, postoperative exercises, and self-care techniques. They provide guidance on mobility aids, assistive devices, and safety precautions to ensure a safe and successful recovery.

Orthopedic nursing requires expertise in musculoskeletal anatomy, surgical techniques, pain management, rehabilitation, and patient teaching. Continuous professional development and staying updated with advancements in orthopedic care are essential for delivering high-quality care to orthopedic patients.

81. Oxygen saturation

Oxygen saturation, often referred to as SpO2 (peripheral oxygen saturation), is a measure of the percentage of hemoglobin in the blood that is saturated with oxygen. In nursing, oxygen saturation is a critical parameter used to assess a patient's respiratory status and adequacy of oxygenation.

Here's what oxygen saturation represents and how it is measured in nursing:

1. Oxygen-binding capacity: Hemoglobin is a protein in red blood cells that carries oxygen throughout the body. Oxygen saturation measures how much of the hemoglobin is bound to oxygen. It indicates the efficiency of oxygen transport in the bloodstream.

2. Non-invasive measurement: Oxygen saturation is typically measured non-invasively using a pulse oximeter. A pulse oximeter is a small device that clips onto a patient's finger, toe, or earlobe. It emits light that passes through the tissue, and it measures the amount of light absorbed by oxygenated and deoxygenated hemoglobin, providing an oxygen saturation reading.

3. Normal range: The normal oxygen saturation level for a healthy individual is usually between 95% and 100%. However, certain factors such as chronic lung disease, heart conditions, or anemia can influence the target range. In some cases, healthcare providers may aim for a slightly lower range to avoid oxygen toxicity.

4. Assessment of respiratory status: Oxygen saturation is an important parameter to assess a patient's respiratory status and evaluate the effectiveness of oxygen therapy

or respiratory interventions. A decrease in oxygen saturation may indicate inadequate oxygenation and potentially signify respiratory distress or compromise.

5. Oxygen therapy management: Nurses play a vital role in managing patients receiving supplemental oxygen therapy. They regularly monitor and document oxygen saturation readings to ensure the prescribed oxygen flow rate provides adequate oxygenation. Based on the oxygen saturation levels, nurses collaborate with the healthcare team to adjust oxygen delivery or escalate care as needed.

Accurate measurement and interpretation of oxygen saturation require proper technique, positioning, and calibration of the pulse oximeter. Nurses should also consider other clinical signs and symptoms alongside oxygen saturation readings to have a comprehensive understanding of a patient's respiratory status.

82. Pneumonia

Pneumonia in nursing refers to the medical condition where there is inflammation of the lungs predominantly caused by infection, resulting in symptoms such as cough, difficulty breathing, chest pain, and fever. In nursing, understanding pneumonia is crucial for the assessment, diagnosis, and management of patients with this respiratory infection.

Here's what pneumonia entails in nursing:

1. Assessment: Nurses perform a comprehensive assessment of patients suspected or diagnosed with pneumonia. This includes assessing the patient's respiratory status, such as the rate and depth of breathing, oxygen saturation levels, and the presence of abnormal lung sounds. Nurses also assess for associated symptoms like fever, cough, sputum production, and chest pain.

2. Diagnosis: In collaboration with the healthcare team, nurses assist in diagnosing pneumonia by relaying patient assessments, vital signs, and other relevant information

to physicians. This may involve documenting signs of infection, abnormal lung sounds, and abnormal chest X-ray findings.

3. Infection control: Nursing plays a critical role in preventing the spread of pneumonia in healthcare settings. This involves adhering to proper infection prevention measures, including hand hygiene, proper personal protective equipment (PPE), and isolation precautions when necessary. Nurses educate patients, families, and colleagues on these infection control practices.

4. Monitoring and treatment: Nurses closely monitor patients with pneumonia, regularly assessing vital signs, oxygen saturation levels, and respiratory status. They administer prescribed medications, such as antibiotics, bronchodilators, and antipyretics, as well as provide supportive care to alleviate symptoms and promote recovery. Nurses also ensure adequate hydration and nutritional support for patients.

5. Patient education: Nurses educate patients and their families about pneumonia, its causes, prevention strategies, and treatment. They provide information on the importance of completing the prescribed course of antibiotics, maintaining good respiratory hygiene, and seeking medical attention if symptoms worsen or don't improve.

6. Collaboration and communication: Nurses collaborate with the healthcare team, including physicians, respiratory therapists, and pharmacists, to develop and implement the most appropriate plan of care for patients with pneumonia. Effective communication ensures timely interventions and continuity of care.

Managing pneumonia requires vigilant monitoring, timely interventions, and patient education. Additionally, nurses play a crucial role in recognizing complications, such as respiratory distress, sepsis, or pleural effusion, and promptly communicating these findings to the appropriate healthcare professionals for further evaluation and management.

83. Poisoning

In nursing, poisoning refers to the ingestion, inhalation, or exposure to harmful substances that can cause detrimental effects on the body. Nurses play a vital role in the assessment, management, and prevention of poisoning cases.

Here's what poisoning entails in nursing:

1. Assessment: Nurses assess patients suspected or known to have been exposed to a poisonous substance. This includes evaluating the patient's signs and symptoms, obtaining a thorough history of the exposure, and assessing vital signs. Nurses also assess the patient's airway, breathing, and circulation to identify any immediate life-threatening complications.

2. Stabilization and emergency care: Nurses provide immediate interventions focused on stabilizing the patient's condition. This may involve ensuring an open airway, assisting with breathing if necessary, providing oxygen, and initiating cardiopulmonary resuscitation (CPR) if the patient is in cardiac arrest. Nurses also administer antidotes or specific treatments as directed by the healthcare team.

3. Monitoring and supportive care: Nurses closely monitor vital signs, oxygen saturation levels, and other relevant parameters to assess the patient's response to treatment and identify any complications. They provide supportive care, such as administering intravenous fluids, medications for symptom management, and implementing measures to maintain the patient's comfort and safety.

4. Collaboration with the healthcare team: Nurses work collaboratively with the healthcare team, including physicians, pharmacists, and toxicologists, to determine the appropriate treatment plan. They communicate relevant information regarding the poisoning, provide updates on the patient's condition, and assist with the implementation of interventions as ordered.

5. Patient education and prevention: Nurses play a crucial role in educating patients and their families about the dangers of poisoning, including potential sources and preventive measures. They provide information on safety precautions, proper storage of medications and toxic substances, and the importance of poison control centers in case of emergencies.

6. Follow-up care and referrals: Nurses may be involved in providing continued care and follow-up for patients who have experienced poisoning. This may include monitoring the patient's progress, providing counseling or mental health support, and referring the patient to appropriate resources for ongoing care or rehabilitation if necessary.

Preventing poisoning incidents is a significant aspect of nursing practice. Nurses contribute to public health efforts by promoting awareness about poisoning risks, participating in community education programs, and advocating for safety measures to reduce the incidence of poisoning.

84. Pulse

In nursing, the term "pulse" refers to the rhythmic expansion and contraction of the arteries as a result of the heart pumping blood throughout the body. Pulse is a vital sign that provides information about the heart rate, rhythm, and strength, allowing healthcare professionals to assess a patient's cardiovascular function.

Here's what pulse entails in nursing:

1. Assessment: Nurses assess the pulse by palpating or feeling the pulsations at various sites in the body where arteries are close to the surface. The most commonly used sites for pulse assessment include the radial artery (wrist), carotid artery (neck), brachial artery (upper arm), and femoral artery (groin). Nurses evaluate the rate (number of beats per minute), rhythm (regular or irregular), and strength (bounding, weak, or thready) of the pulse.

2. Vital sign: Pulse is considered one of the important vital signs alongside temperature, blood pressure, and respiratory rate. It provides valuable information about the patient's overall cardiovascular health and can help identify underlying conditions or changes in the body's physiology.

3. Cardiac output and perfusion: Pulse reflects the function of the heart as it pumps blood to deliver oxygen and nutrients to the body's tissues and organs. Changes in the pulse rate or quality can indicate alterations in cardiac output or perfusion. Increased pulse rate may suggest factors such as stress, exercise, fever, or cardiovascular conditions. Decreased pulse rate, on the other hand, may indicate issues such as bradycardia, medication effects, or conditions affecting cardiac function.

4. Monitoring during interventions: Nurses frequently assess the patient's pulse before, during, and after interventions, such as administering medication, blood transfusions, or during invasive procedures. Monitoring the pulse helps ensure patient safety, identify any adverse reactions, and assess the patient's response to treatment or interventions.

5. Documentation and communication: Accurate documentation of pulse rate, rhythm, and other relevant findings is essential in nursing. Nurses document the pulse rate along with other vital signs, observations, and pertinent information in the patient's medical record. They also communicate the patient's pulse status to other healthcare team members in handover reports or interdisciplinary discussions for continuity of care.

Assessing the pulse requires trained palpation skills and familiarity with normal and abnormal findings. Nurses must consider factors that can affect pulse, including age, fitness level, medication use, and underlying health conditions. Regular monitoring of pulse is a fundamental part of nursing practice, aiding in the evaluation of cardiovascular status, detecting abnormalities, and guiding patient care decisions.

85. QD (once daily)

In nursing, "QD" is an abbreviation derived from the Latin phrase "quaque die," which means "once daily." It is commonly used to denote the frequency or dosing schedule of medication administration. When a medication order specifies QD, it means that the medication should be taken once a day.

Here's what QD (once daily) means in nursing:

1. Medication administration: When a medication order instructs "QD" or "once daily," it indicates that the medication should be given to the patient once every 24 hours. Typically, the time of day for medication administration may be specified, or healthcare providers may specify a preferred time based on factors such as drug absorption, therapeutic effect, or patient preference.

2. Dosing schedule: QD dosing is commonly used for medications where a once-daily dosing regimen is deemed appropriate and effective. Some medications, especially those with an extended-release formulation, are designed to release the drug slowly over a prolonged period, allowing for a once-daily dosing schedule.

3. Compliance and medication adherence: QD dosing can simplify medication regimens and enhance patient compliance and adherence to the prescribed treatment. Taking medications only once a day can be more convenient and easier to remember, particularly for patients who struggle with complex medication schedules or have difficulty managing multiple doses throughout the day.

4. Patient education: Nurses play a crucial role in educating patients about their medications and dosing schedules. When a medication is prescribed QD, nurses explain to patients when and how to take the medication. They provide instructions on the importance of taking the medication consistently at the same time each day and emphasize the need to complete the full prescribed course of treatment.

It's important to note that medication orders and abbreviations must be carefully interpreted and clearly communicated to avoid medication errors. In healthcare practice, it is necessary to adhere to strict guidelines and policies regarding abbreviations. Nurses should always refer to their organization's approved list of abbreviations and clarify any uncertainties with prescribers or pharmacists.

86. QID (four times daily)

In nursing, "QID" is an abbreviation derived from the Latin phrase "quater in die," which means "four times daily." It is commonly used to indicate the frequency or dosing schedule of medication administration. When a medication order specifies QID, it means that the medication should be taken four times a day at regular intervals.

Here's what QID (four times daily) means in nursing:

1. Medication administration: When a medication order instructs "QID" or "four times daily," it indicates that the medication should be given to the patient four times over a 24-hour period. The times at which the medication should be administered are typically specified by the healthcare provider based on factors such as drug absorption, therapeutic effect, or patient needs.

2. Dosing schedule: QID dosing is commonly used for medications that require frequent administration throughout the day to maintain therapeutic levels in the body. Examples may include medications with a short half-life or those requiring more frequent dose adjustments or titration.

3. Compliance and medication adherence: QID dosing can present challenges for patients in terms of medication adherence and compliance. Taking medications four times daily may be more difficult to remember and manage, particularly for patients with complex medication regimens or those who have difficulty adhering to strict timing requirements. Nurses play a crucial role in educating and supporting patients to ensure they understand and can adhere to the prescribed dosing schedule.

4. Patient education: Nurses are responsible for educating patients about their medications and dosing schedules. When a medication is prescribed QID, nurses provide instructions on when and how to take the medication. They explain the importance of taking the medication at the specified times, emphasizing adherence and the completion of the full prescribed course of treatment.

It is important for nurses to ensure clear and accurate communication of medication orders and dosing schedules. They should reference their organization's approved list of abbreviations and seek clarification from the prescriber or pharmacist when necessary. Adherence to proper medication administration practices and patient education is crucial to prevent errors and optimize medication outcomes.

87. Radiography

Radiography in nursing refers to the use of medical imaging techniques, such as X-rays, to create images of the internal structures of the body. Nurses may be involved in various aspects of radiography, including preparation of patients, assisting during the procedure, and interpreting and utilizing the images for patient care.

Here's what radiography entails in nursing:

1. Patient preparation: Nurses play a role in preparing patients for radiographic procedures. This may involve explaining the procedure, obtaining informed consent, assessing the patient for any contraindications or allergies to contrast agents, and providing instructions on any necessary preparations (such as fasting or removal of jewelry or clothing).

2. Assisting during the procedure: Nurses may assist the radiologic technologist or radiographer during the radiographic examination. This can include positioning the patient correctly, ensuring proper shielding for radiation safety, providing support and reassurance to the patient, and assisting with any necessary equipment or instrumentation.

3. Image interpretation: While nurses are not typically responsible for interpreting radiographic images themselves, they often collaborate with radiologists and other healthcare professionals to analyze and interpret the findings. Nurses may need to understand basic radiographic concepts and terminology to effectively communicate with the radiology team and incorporate the imaging results into patient care plans.

4. Utilizing images for patient care: Once radiographic images are obtained, nurses may use them as part of their assessment and care planning. They may review the images to identify and document any abnormalities or changes in the patient's condition. Nurses may also monitor and assess the patient for any adverse reactions to contrast agents or radiation exposure and provide appropriate nursing interventions and support.

5. Patient education: Nurses have a vital role in providing patient education related to radiography. This may include explaining the purpose and benefits of the procedure, discussing any potential risks or discomfort, and addressing any concerns or questions the patient may have.

Nurses collaborate with the radiology department and the broader healthcare team to ensure the safe and effective use of radiographic techniques for diagnostic and therapeutic purposes. They must adhere to established protocols, maintain patient safety, and effectively communicate and document imaging findings to facilitate optimal patient care.

88. Respiration

In nursing, respiration refers to the process of breathing and the exchange of oxygen and carbon dioxide in the body. It is an essential physiological function that supplies oxygen to the cells and removes carbon dioxide to maintain the body's acid-base balance.

Here's what respiration entails in nursing:

1. Assessment: Nurses assess a patient's respiration by evaluating various components. This includes monitoring the rate of breathing (respiratory rate), assessing the depth and effort of breathing, and observing for any abnormalities in the pattern or rhythm of breaths. They also assess the patient's oxygen saturation levels using a pulse oximeter to determine the adequacy of oxygenation.

2. Respiratory interventions: Nurses provide interventions and support to promote effective respiration. This may involve assisting with positioning for optimal lung expansion, ensuring a clear airway, administering supplemental oxygen, or administering medications to relieve respiratory distress or reduce inflammation in the airways. Nurses may also initiate or assist with respiratory treatments such as nebulizer therapy or chest physiotherapy.

3. Monitoring and management of devices: In some situations, patients may require assistance with respiratory function through the use of devices such as ventilators, continuous positive airway pressure (CPAP), or bi-level positive airway pressure (BiPAP). Nurses monitor these devices, assess the patient's response and comfort, and maintain the proper functioning of the equipment.

4. Patient education: Nurses play a crucial role in educating patients and their families about respiratory health and management. This can include teaching proper breathing techniques, explaining the importance of deep breathing and coughing to prevent complications such as pneumonia, and providing guidance on smoking cessation to improve respiratory function.

5. Collaboration and referral: Nurses collaborate with the healthcare team, such as respiratory therapists or physicians, to ensure comprehensive respiratory care for patients. They communicate any changes in respiratory status, seek appropriate consultations or referrals, and contribute to the development and implementation of a plan of care.

Respiration is a vital aspect of nursing care, and accurate assessment and management of respiratory function are crucial for patients' overall health and well-being. By maintaining respiratory health, preventing complications, and promoting effective breathing, nurses help patients optimize oxygenation and maintain optimal functioning of the respiratory system.

89. Rehabilitation

In nursing, rehabilitation refers to the process of helping individuals recover, regain independence, and improve their physical, cognitive, and functional abilities after an illness, injury, or surgery. Rehabilitation nursing focuses on providing comprehensive care and support to patients throughout their rehabilitation journey.

Here's what rehabilitation entails in nursing:

1. Assessment: Nurses conduct thorough assessments to evaluate the patient's physical, cognitive, and psychosocial functioning. This includes assessing mobility, strength, coordination, balance, cognition, communication, and emotional well-being. Nurses also assess the patient's goals, preferences, and readiness for rehabilitation.

2. Care planning: Based on the assessment findings, nurses collaborate with the healthcare team, including rehabilitation specialists and therapists, to develop a personalized care plan. This plan outlines the goals, interventions, and strategies to optimize the patient's recovery and functional outcomes. Nurses play a crucial role in continuity of care by ensuring that the plan is communicated effectively to other team members.

3. Rehabilitation interventions: Nurses implement a variety of rehabilitation interventions to support the patient's recovery. These can include assisting with activities of daily living (ADLs), providing mobility assistance and training, administering and monitoring prescribed medications, managing pain and discomfort,

promoting proper nutrition and hydration, and facilitating communication and cognitive exercises.

4. Patient and family education: Nurses educate patients and their families about the rehabilitation process, goals, and expectations. They provide information on techniques for safe and independent mobility, strategies for managing symptoms and preventing complications, and practical tips for adapting the home environment to promote a safe and supportive recovery. Education also includes preparing patients and families for discharge and providing resources for ongoing rehabilitation needs.

5. Emotional support and counseling: Nurses provide emotional support and counseling to patients and families throughout the rehabilitation process. They understand the emotional challenges and potential psychological impact associated with significant health changes. Nurses offer empathy, encouragement, and guidance, helping patients and families cope with their emotions and navigate the rehabilitation journey.

6. Collaboration and coordination: Rehabilitation nursing involves close collaboration and coordination with various members of the healthcare team, including physical therapists, occupational therapists, speech-language pathologists, social workers, and psychologists. Nurses actively engage in rehabilitation team meetings, care conferences, and interdisciplinary communication to ensure continuity and effectiveness of care.

Rehabilitation nursing aims to promote independence, enhance quality of life, and empower individuals to reach their fullest potential during the recovery process. It requires compassion, clinical expertise, and effective communication skills to support patients and their families in achieving meaningful rehabilitation outcomes.

90. Scalpel

Scalpel is a surgical instrument used by healthcare professionals, including nurses, during medical procedures. It consists of a small, sharp blade attached to a handle. Nurses may use a scalpel under the supervision of a surgeon or physician to make precise incisions during surgeries or other medical interventions.

91. Sepsis

Sepsis is a potentially life-threatening condition that can occur when the body's response to an infection causes widespread inflammation throughout the body. In nursing, sepsis refers to the recognition, assessment, and management of patients who are at risk or have developed sepsis. Nurses play a crucial role in identifying early signs and symptoms of sepsis, such as increased heart rate, altered mental status, fever, and low blood pressure. They also monitor patients closely and initiate appropriate interventions, such as administering antibiotics and fluids, to help prevent the progression of sepsis and maintain patient stability.

92. Serology

In nursing, serology refers to the study and analysis of blood serum for the detection of specific antibodies or antigens. It involves laboratory testing of blood samples to identify and diagnose infectious diseases, immune responses, and certain medical conditions. Serology tests are commonly used to detect antibodies produced by the body's immune system in response to an infection or to determine if an individual has been previously exposed to a particular pathogen. Nurses may collect blood samples from patients and work in collaboration with laboratory professionals to interpret and utilize serology test results in the diagnosis and management of patients' health conditions.

93. Shock

In nursing, shock refers to a life-threatening condition where there is inadequate blood flow reaching the organs and tissues of the body. It is typically caused by a severe drop in blood pressure, resulting in reduced oxygen and nutrient supply to various parts of the body.

Nurses play a critical role in the recognition, assessment, and management of shock. They closely monitor vital signs, such as blood pressure, heart rate, and oxygen saturation levels, to identify signs of shock. Prompt interventions, including administering intravenous fluids, providing oxygen therapy, and initiating medications to support blood pressure, are initiated by nurses.

Furthermore, nurses must also address the underlying cause of shock, such as hemorrhage, infection, or anaphylaxis, in collaboration with the healthcare team. The goal is to stabilize the patient's condition, optimize organ perfusion, and restore normal blood pressure to prevent organ damage and improve patient outcomes.

94. Sore throat

In nursing, a sore throat refers to discomfort, pain, or irritation in the throat, often accompanied by difficulty swallowing, inflammation, and sometimes swollen tonsils. It can be caused by various factors, including viral or bacterial infections, allergies, or irritants like smoke.

Nurses play a role in assessing and managing patients with sore throats. They gather the patient's medical history, including symptoms and duration, and perform a physical examination to evaluate the severity of the condition. Nurses may use tools such as a throat swab to collect a specimen for laboratory analysis to determine the cause of the sore throat, especially if a bacterial infection, such as strep throat, is suspected.

Treatment approaches for a sore throat can include symptomatic relief measures such as over-the-counter pain relievers, warm liquids, throat lozenges, or soothing gargles. If a bacterial infection is present, nurses may assist with administering prescribed antibiotics and educating the patient about adherence to the treatment regimen.

Furthermore, nurses provide patient education on self-care management, including rest, hydration, and avoiding irritants, to support recovery and alleviate symptoms.

95. Specimen

In nursing, a specimen refers to a sample of body fluid, tissue, or other biological material that is collected from a patient for diagnostic testing or analysis. Specimens are used to identify and diagnose various conditions, monitor disease progression, and guide treatment decisions.

Nurses play a vital role in specimen collection, handling, and documentation. They are responsible for ensuring proper identification of the patient and specimen, maintaining sterile technique during the collection process, and adhering to infection control protocols. Common types of specimens collected by nurses may include blood, urine, sputum, wound swabs, or throat swabs.

Additionally, nurses may assist with labeling, packaging, and transporting the specimens to the laboratory for further analysis. It is crucial for nurses to accurately document the collection details, including the date, time, and method used, as well as any relevant patient information, to ensure proper tracking and interpretation of results. Effective specimen management is essential to provide accurate and timely information for patient care.

96. Stethoscope

A stethoscope is a medical device that is used by nurses and other healthcare professionals to listen to the internal sounds of a patient's body. It consists of a chest piece attached to tubing, which connects to earpieces worn by the healthcare professional. The chest piece is placed on different areas of the patient's body, such as the chest, back, or abdomen, to capture sounds like heartbeats, breathing sounds, and bowel sounds. Nurses use the stethoscope to assess the health status of patients and to monitor their heart and lung functions. It is an essential tool in nursing for conducting physical examinations and diagnosing various conditions.

97. Stool

In nursing, "stool" refers to the waste material that is excreted from the body during a bowel movement or defecation. It is also known as feces or bowel motion. Nurses often monitor and assess the characteristics of a patient's stool as it can provide important information about their digestive and overall health. This includes observing the color, consistency, frequency, and odor of the stool. Changes in stool characteristics may indicate various conditions or disorders, such as gastrointestinal infections, inflammation, bleeding, or malabsorption issues. Nurses may collect stool samples for laboratory analysis to aid in diagnosing and treating certain conditions.

98. Stroke

In nursing, "stroke" refers to a medical condition known as a cerebrovascular accident (CVA). A stroke occurs when there is a disruption of blood flow to a part of the brain, leading to damage or death of brain cells. Nurses play a crucial role in the care and management of stroke patients.

In the context of nursing, stroke refers to:

1. Assessment: Nurses are responsible for assessing and monitoring patients who have had a stroke. This includes assessing vital signs, neurological status, level of consciousness, motor function, speech, and cognitive abilities.

2. Acute care: Nurses are involved in the acute care of stroke patients, ensuring that they receive immediate medical intervention, such as thrombolytic therapy (if appropriate) to dissolve blood clots. They also monitor and manage potential complications, such as respiratory distress, bleeding, or cardiac issues.

3. Rehabilitation: Nursing care in stroke includes assisting with the rehabilitation process. Nurses may help patients with activities of daily living (ADLs), mobility exercises, and speech therapy. They also educate patients and their families on stroke prevention, lifestyle modifications, and medications.

4. Medication administration: Nurses may administer medications, such as antiplatelet agents or anticoagulants, to prevent further strokes or manage associated conditions like hypertension or diabetes.

5. Emotional support: Stroke patients may experience emotional and psychological challenges. Nurses provide emotional support, counseling, and education to both patients and their families to help them cope with the physical and emotional effects of stroke.

The role of nursing in stroke care involves interdisciplinary collaboration with other healthcare professionals to ensure comprehensive and holistic care for stroke patients.

99. Subcutaneous

In nursing, "subcutaneous" (often abbreviated as "subQ" or "SQ") refers to a route of medication administration or a type of tissue.

1. Subcutaneous (route of medication administration): Subcutaneous administration involves delivering medication into the fatty tissue layer just beneath the skin. The medication is typically injected using a small needle or administered through an insulin pen or an autoinjector device. Examples of medications commonly given subcutaneously include insulin, anticoagulants (such as heparin), certain vaccines, and hormone therapies. Nurses often administer subcutaneous injections to patients, taking care to choose appropriate injection sites, rotate sites to prevent tissue irritation, and ensure proper dosage and technique.

2. Subcutaneous (tissue): Subcutaneous tissue, also known as the hypodermis, is the layer of tissue found beneath the dermis and above the muscle. It is composed of fat cells and connective tissue that insulate, protect, and provide a cushioning effect. In nursing, knowledge of the subcutaneous tissue is important when administering medications, such as subcutaneous injections, and when assessing wounds or

performing procedures, such as the placement of subcutaneous sutures or the insertion of subcutaneous implants or devices.

Understanding subcutaneous administration and the subcutaneous tissue is essential for nurses to provide safe and effective care for their patients. It is important to follow the proper protocols and guidelines to ensure accurate medication administration and minimize adverse effects.

100. Surgery

In nursing, "surgery" refers to a specialized field of healthcare involving medical procedures that involve incisions or manipulations of bodily tissues to treat or diagnose a condition. Nurses play vital roles in various aspects of surgical care, assisting before, during, and after the surgical procedure.

In the context of nursing, surgery includes:

1. Preoperative care: Nurses are involved in the preoperative phase, which begins before the actual surgery. They assess the patient's medical history, perform physical examinations, and conduct necessary diagnostic tests. They also educate patients about the upcoming surgery, provide instructions for preoperative preparations (such as fasting or medication restrictions), and address any concerns or questions the patient may have.

2. Intraoperative care: Nurses support the surgical team during the operation. They are responsible for ensuring the operating room is adequately prepared with necessary equipment, maintaining sterile principles, and assisting the surgeon and other team members in various tasks. They monitor the patient's vital signs, administer medications as directed, anticipate the surgeon's needs, and maintain documentation and record-keeping.

3. Postoperative care: Nurses provide postoperative care to patients recovering from surgery. This includes closely monitoring vital signs, assessing the patient's pain level,

managing wound care, administering medications (such as pain relievers or antibiotics), and monitoring for potential complications. Nurses also educate patients and their families on postoperative care instructions, potential side effects, and signs of complications that may occur after surgery.

4. Advocacy and support: Nurses act as advocates for patients undergoing surgery, ensuring their safety, comfort, and well-being. They provide emotional support, address any concerns or anxieties, and facilitate communication between the patient and the surgical team. Nurses also play a crucial role in patient education, helping patients understand their procedures, promoting informed decision-making, and ensuring they have the necessary information to care for themselves postoperatively.

Nursing in the surgical setting requires a wide range of skills, including technical competence, critical thinking, effective communication, and attention to detail. Nurses work closely with other members of the surgical team, such as surgeons, anesthesiologists, and surgical technologists, to provide optimal patient care and contribute to successful surgical outcomes.

101. Suture

In nursing, a "suture" refers to a medical stitch or thread that is used to close a wound or incision. Suturing is a common procedure performed by nurses, particularly those working in surgical units, emergency departments, or wound care clinics.

When a patient has a wound that requires closure, nurses may use sutures to bring the edges of the wound together and facilitate the healing process. Sutures are typically made of a sterile, thread-like material, such as nylon or polypropylene, that is strong and biocompatible.

Nurses who are trained in suturing techniques are responsible for:

1. Preparation: Prior to suturing, nurses prepare the necessary supplies, including sterile instruments, suture materials, and local anesthetic if needed. They ensure the area around the wound is properly cleaned and prepped to minimize the risk of infection.

2. Suture selection: Nurses choose the appropriate type and size of suture based on factors such as the size and location of the wound, the tension on the wound edges, and the patient's individual needs. Different types of sutures, such as absorbable or non-absorbable sutures, may be used depending on the specific wound characteristics.

3. Suturing technique: Nurses utilize their knowledge of suturing techniques to close the wound effectively. This may involve using various suturing methods, such as simple interrupted sutures, continuous sutures, or running subcuticular sutures. Nurses must ensure that the wound edges are properly aligned and that the sutures are placed with precision and appropriate tension.

4. Wound care: After suturing, nurses educate the patient on proper wound care and provide instructions for activities to avoid, signs of infection, and when to have the sutures removed or follow-up with a healthcare provider.

In addition to suturing wounds, nurses may also be involved in removing sutures or staples at the appropriate time during the healing process. Proper suture removal techniques help ensure patient comfort and minimize the risk of complications or scarring.

Overall, suturing is an essential skill for nurses involved in wound management, surgical care, or emergency procedures, allowing them to contribute to the healing process and promote positive patient outcomes.

102. Swab

In nursing, a "swab" refers to a small piece of absorbent material, such as cotton or gauze, that is used to collect samples, apply medication, or clean a specific area during various medical procedures.

Here are a few common uses of swabs in nursing:

1. Sample collection: Nurses may use swabs to collect samples from different body sites, such as the throat, nasal passages, wound sites, or genital areas. These samples can be sent to the laboratory for analysis to help diagnose infections or other medical conditions.

2. Wound care: Swabs can be employed to clean wounds or apply topical medications, such as antiseptics or dressings. Nurses may use sterile swabs to gently wipe or remove debris from the wound site, aiding in the healing process and preventing infection.

3. Specimen application: Swabs are used to apply substances or medications to specific areas. For instance, during a medical procedure or examination, a nurse may use a swab to apply anesthetic gel to numb a targeted region before an injection or procedure.

4. Sterility maintenance: In sterile procedures, nurses may utilize swabs for purposes such as wiping down the skin before insertion of an intravenous catheter or cleaning an area before a surgical incision. Swabs help maintain a sterile environment by removing surface contaminants and reducing the risk of infection.

Nurses must adhere to strict guidelines when using swabs to ensure patient safety and prevent cross-contamination. This includes using sterile swabs for sterile procedures, handling swabs in a manner that prevents contamination, and properly disposing of used swabs after their intended use.

Overall, swabs are versatile tools used by nurses to perform various functions like sample collection, wound care, medication application, and maintaining sterility in medical procedures.

103. Syringe

In nursing, a syringe refers to a medical device that is used for administering medications, fluids, or other substances into the body or extracting bodily fluids for testing or analysis. A syringe typically consists of a hollow barrel, a plunger, and a needle. Nurses often use syringes to administer medications through injections or other routes such as intravenous, intramuscular, or subcutaneous. Syringes come in different sizes, depending on the volume of medication or fluid to be administered.

104. Tamponade

In nursing, tamponade refers to a medical condition known as cardiac tamponade. It occurs when there is a build-up of fluid or blood in the space around the heart, called the pericardial sac. The increased pressure from the fluid compresses the heart, preventing it from filling and pumping blood effectively.

Nurses play a crucial role in identifying and managing tamponade. They monitor patients for signs and symptoms such as chest pain, shortness of breath, low blood pressure, rapid heart rate, and decreased urine output. When tamponade is suspected, nurses collaborate with healthcare providers to perform diagnostic tests, like echocardiography and cardiac catheterization, to confirm the diagnosis.

Immediate intervention is necessary to relieve the pressure on the heart in cases of tamponade. Nurses may provide supportive care, such as administering oxygen and medications to stabilize the patient. Depending on the severity of the condition, procedures like pericardiocentesis or pericardial window may be performed to drain the fluid and alleviate the tamponade. Nurses closely monitor patients following intervention to ensure their condition improves and to prevent any complications.

105. Telemetry

In nursing, telemetry refers to the continuous monitoring of a patient's vital signs and cardiac activity, usually done remotely. Telemetry involves the use of electronic devices called telemetry monitors, which are connected to the patient through electrodes or sensors.

Telemetry monitors continuously measure and transmit data about the patient's heart rate, rhythm, blood pressure, oxygen saturation level, and other parameters. This information is displayed on a central monitoring station, where nurses and other healthcare professionals can observe and analyze the patient's condition in real-time.

Telemetry is particularly useful for patients who require close monitoring, such as those recovering from cardiac procedures, experiencing heart-related conditions, or in critical care units. It allows nurses to detect any abnormalities or changes in the patient's vital signs promptly and respond accordingly.

In addition to monitoring, nurses are responsible for interpreting the telemetry data, recognizing patterns or potential complications, and taking appropriate actions. They may adjust medications, notify the healthcare team of any concerning findings, or intervene if the patient's condition deteriorates. Nurses also ensure that the telemetry equipment is properly functioning and electrodes are correctly placed and secured for accurate readings.

106. Thoracotomy

In nursing, thoracotomy refers to a surgical procedure in which an incision is made into the chest wall to access the organs within the thoracic cavity. It is a major surgical intervention that is performed by healthcare providers, such as surgeons, to treat various conditions or perform certain diagnostic procedures.

Thoracotomy allows access to the lungs, heart, esophagus, and other structures within the chest. It may be done to remove tumors, repair injured organs, treat lung infections, manage complications of trauma, or diagnose certain conditions. The specific approach and extent of the incision depend on the purpose of the procedure and the patient's medical condition.

Nurses play a crucial role in caring for patients who undergo thoracotomy. They provide preoperative assessments and education, ensuring that patients are well-informed and prepared for the procedure. During the surgery, nurses are responsible for assisting in the sterile setup, providing instruments and supplies, and maintaining the patient's safety and comfort.

Postoperatively, nurses closely monitor the patient's vital signs, assess for any signs of complications, and provide appropriate pain management. They assist with wound care, respiratory treatments, and mobilization. As the patient recovers, nurses educate and support them and their family in the management of postoperative pain, medications, breathing exercises, and wound healing.

Nurses also play a vital role in monitoring and managing potential complications that can arise after a thoracotomy, such as infections, bleeding, breathing difficulties, or complications related to anesthesia. They collaborate with the healthcare team to ensure a smooth recovery and provide comprehensive care throughout the entire process.

107. Tincture

In nursing, a tincture refers to a medication that is prepared by dissolving a drug in an alcohol or alcohol-water mixture. Tinctures are typically used for oral administration, and the alcohol acts as a solvent to extract the active components of the drug. Tinctures are commonly used for herbal medications or natural remedies.

108. Transfusion

In nursing, a transfusion refers to the process of infusing blood or blood products into a patient's bloodstream. This is done to replace lost blood components, such as red blood cells, platelets, or plasma, or to provide specific elements such as clotting factors or antibodies. Transfusions are carried out when a patient's blood volume or specific blood components are deficient due to conditions such as blood loss, surgery, anemia, or certain medical treatments. Nurses play a crucial role in ensuring the safe administration of transfusions by verifying compatibility, monitoring the patient's vital signs, and assessing for any adverse reactions.

109. Trauma

In nursing, trauma refers to a severe physical injury or wound sustained by a patient. Trauma can result from accidents, falls, violence, or other incidents that cause significant damage to the body. Traumatic injuries can affect various body systems and may include fractures, lacerations, burns, internal injuries, or head injuries. Nurses who specialize in trauma care or work in an emergency department are trained to provide immediate and comprehensive care to patients with trauma. This includes assessing and stabilizing the patient's condition, managing pain, administering medications or intravenous fluids, monitoring vital signs, and coordinating further diagnostic tests or interventions, such as surgery. Additionally, nurses play a critical role in providing emotional support to patients and their families during the traumatic event and throughout the recovery process.

110. Triage

In nursing, triage refers to the systematic process of assessing and prioritizing patients based on the severity of their condition or injury. Triage is commonly used in emergency departments, clinics, or disaster situations where there may be limited resources or a large number of patients needing care. The goal of triage is to determine which patients require immediate medical attention and which can wait or may have a lower acuity level.

During triage, nurses use a standardized system to quickly evaluate patients' vital signs, symptoms, and level of distress. The patients are then categorized into different priority levels, typically designated as immediate, urgent, non-urgent, or expectant. This allows healthcare providers to allocate resources efficiently and provide immediate care to those with the greatest need.

Nurses in a triage role must possess strong assessment skills, critical thinking abilities, and the ability to make rapid decisions. They also need good communication skills to effectively communicate with patients, their families, and other members of the healthcare team to ensure appropriate and timely care is provided.

111. Ultrasound

In nursing, ultrasound refers to the use of high-frequency sound waves to create images of the internal structures of the body. Ultrasound technology is non-invasive and uses a handheld device called a transducer, which emits sound waves that are reflected back to create real-time images.

In nursing, ultrasound is commonly used for diagnostic purposes to assess organs, tissues, and blood vessels. For example, it can be used to evaluate the condition of the heart, liver, kidneys, or uterus, and identify any abnormalities or diseases.

Ultrasound is also used in obstetrics for monitoring the development and health of the fetus during pregnancy. It allows nurses to visualize the fetal anatomy, determine the gestational age, and assess the well-being of the baby.

Nurses who specialize in ultrasound, known as ultrasound technicians or sonographers, perform the procedure under the guidance of a physician. They play a critical role in positioning the patient, applying gel to the skin for better sound wave transmission, and operating the ultrasound equipment to obtain clear and accurate images. Nurses may also assist with interpreting the ultrasound results and collaborating with the healthcare team to develop an appropriate care plan for the patient.

112. Urinalysis

In nursing, urinalysis refers to the laboratory examination and analysis of urine. It involves the testing of a urine sample to detect and evaluate various substances, including chemical compounds, cells, and organisms present in the urine.

Urinalysis is a commonly performed diagnostic test that provides valuable information about a person's health and helps in the diagnosis and monitoring of various conditions. It can help identify urinary tract infections, kidney diseases, diabetes, liver disorders, and other medical conditions.

Nurses play a crucial role in collecting urine samples from patients, ensuring proper labeling and storage, and providing instructions on how to obtain a clean catch or midstream sample. They may also perform some basic physical and visual examinations of the urine specimen, such as checking its color, clarity, and odor. Nurses may also assist in transporting the urine samples to the laboratory and communicate the results to the healthcare team for further analysis and interpretation.

113. Vaccination

In nursing, vaccination refers to the administration of vaccines to individuals in order to prevent specific infectious diseases. Vaccination involves the introduction of a vaccine into the body to stimulate the immune system and produce protection against a particular disease-causing organism (pathogen) such as viruses or bacteria.

Nurses play a crucial role in the process of vaccination. This includes assessing the patient's medical history and eligibility for vaccination, educating patients and their families about the benefits and potential side effects of vaccines, administering the vaccine by following proper techniques and protocols, and documenting the vaccination in the patient's medical records.

Nurses also monitor patients for any adverse reactions following vaccination and provide appropriate care or guidance if needed. They may be involved in vaccine storage and management, as well as participating in vaccine education campaigns to promote vaccine compliance and public health.

Vaccination is an essential component of preventive healthcare and plays a significant role in reducing the incidence and spread of infectious diseases. It is considered a cost-effective and life-saving intervention, protecting both individuals and communities.

114. Vascular

In nursing, vascular refers to anything related to the blood vessels in the body. This includes the arteries, veins, and capillaries that transport blood throughout the circulatory system.

Nurses who work in vascular care or vascular nursing specialize in the assessment, management, and treatment of vascular conditions and diseases. They may work in various healthcare settings, including hospitals, clinics, specialized vascular centers, or surgical units.

Nurses in vascular care play a crucial role in providing care to patients with vascular conditions such as peripheral artery disease (PAD), deep vein thrombosis (DVT), varicose veins, or vascular injuries. They assess patients' vascular health, monitor for signs of complications, and provide interventions to promote blood flow and prevent further damage.

Nurses may assist in procedures related to vascular access, such as inserting and maintaining intravenous (IV) lines, central venous catheters, or arterial lines. They also educate patients about preventing vascular diseases, managing risk factors, following medication regimens, and lifestyle modifications. In addition, nurses may collaborate with the healthcare team, including vascular surgeons, interventional radiologists, or vascular technicians, to ensure comprehensive and coordinated care for patients with vascular conditions.

115. Venipuncture

In nursing, venipuncture refers to the process of puncturing a vein with a needle to obtain a blood sample or administer intravenous (IV) therapy. It is a common nursing skill used to collect blood for laboratory testing, establish vascular access, or deliver medications or fluids directly into the bloodstream.

Venipuncture involves identifying an appropriate vein, usually in the arm, and using a sterile needle to puncture through the skin and into the vein. The nurse carefully collects the desired amount of blood into a collection tube or prepares the site for the insertion of an IV catheter. After completing the procedure, the nurse properly labels and transports the blood sample to the laboratory for analysis or secures the IV catheter for ongoing therapy.

Nurses are trained in venipuncture techniques to ensure a safe and effective procedure. They follow standard precautions, practice good hand hygiene, and take measures to prevent infection and minimize patient discomfort. Nurses must have a thorough understanding of anatomy, knowledge of different types of veins, and proficiency in the equipment and techniques used for venipuncture. They must also possess good communication and patient care skills, as well as the ability to accurately label and document the collected blood samples.

Venipuncture is an important nursing skill as it enables healthcare professionals to obtain essential diagnostic information, monitor patient conditions, and administer necessary treatments.

116. Ventilation

In nursing, ventilation refers to the process of assisting or supporting a patient's breathing. It involves the delivery of oxygen and the removal of carbon dioxide to maintain adequate oxygenation and ventilation in the body.

Nurses may be involved in various aspects of ventilation, depending on the patient's condition and the level of support required. This can range from simple measures such as providing oxygen therapy through nasal cannula or face mask, to more advanced techniques such as mechanical ventilation using a ventilator.

Nurses monitor the patient's respiratory status, assess breathing patterns, and implement appropriate interventions to support ventilation. They may collaborate with the healthcare team to adjust oxygen flow rates, administer medications to improve lung function, or provide airway clearance techniques to remove secretions and improve ventilation. Nurses also play a significant role in educating patients and their families on proper breathing techniques, the use of respiratory devices, and self-management of respiratory conditions.

In critical care settings or in cases where a patient is unable to breathe adequately on their own, nurses with specialized training may operate and manage mechanical ventilators. This involves ensuring proper settings, monitoring vital signs, assessing lung function, and making adjustments as necessary to optimize ventilation.

Overall, ventilation in nursing aims to ensure the delivery and exchange of gases in the respiratory system, keeping patients well-oxygenated and supporting their breathing efforts.

117. Vitals

In nursing, vitals refer to the essential signs and measurements that provide information about a patient's overall physiological functioning. These vital signs are routinely assessed and monitored to evaluate a patient's health status and detect any potential changes or abnormalities.

The four main vital signs consistently measured in nursing are:

1. Temperature: This is the measurement of a patient's body heat or thermal state. Temperature can be taken orally, rectally, under the armpit, or in the ear.

2. Pulse or Heart Rate: This indicates the rate at which the heart beats per minute. The pulse can be measured at various sites on the body, but the most common locations are the radial artery (wrist) or the carotid artery (neck).

3. Blood Pressure: This measures the force exerted by blood against the walls of the arteries. It is recorded as two numbers – systolic pressure (the higher number) and diastolic pressure (the lower number).

4. Respiratory Rate: This reflects the number of breaths a patient takes per minute. It is counted by observing the rise and fall of the chest or by listening to the patient's breathing sounds.

In addition to these four vital signs, other measurements such as oxygen saturation (SpO2), which indicates the amount of oxygen in the blood, may also be included as a vital sign. Pain assessment is another important aspect of nursing care but is considered a subjective measure.

Nurses regularly assess and document vital signs to establish a baseline, monitor changes, identify trends, and aid in decision-making regarding patient care. Vital signs provide important information about a patient's cardiovascular function, respiratory status, and overall well-being. Monitoring vital signs allows nurses to detect early signs of deterioration or improvement, guide interventions, and evaluate the effectiveness of interventions or treatments.

118. Wound

In nursing, a wound refers to an injury or break in the skin or underlying tissues. Wounds can result from various causes, including trauma, surgical procedures, chronic conditions, or medical treatments.

Nurses play a significant role in the assessment, management, and care of wounds. This includes evaluating the wound's characteristics, such as its size, depth, presence of infection, and degree of healing. Nurses also assess patients' overall health status, risk factors, and any underlying conditions that may impact wound healing.

Nurses are responsible for cleaning and dressing wounds appropriately using sterile techniques to prevent infection and promote healing. They may also apply topical medications, such as antimicrobial ointments or advanced wound dressings, based on the wound's needs.

Monitoring and documenting the wound's progress, as well as assessing for any signs of complications, such as increased pain, redness, swelling, or drainage, are important nursing responsibilities. Nurses also educate patients and caregivers on wound care techniques, signs of infection, and preventive measures, such as proper nutrition, hydration, and regular position changes to prevent pressure ulcers.

In complex or non-healing wounds, nurses may collaborate with other healthcare professionals, such as wound care specialists, surgeons, or physical therapists, to develop a comprehensive care plan. They also play a vital role in providing emotional support to patients, as wounds can be painful and may impact a person's overall well-being.

119. X-ray

In nursing, an X-ray refers to a medical imaging technique that uses ionizing radiation to produce images of the internal structures of the body. X-rays are commonly used for diagnostic purposes to identify fractures, dislocations, lung conditions, infections, abdominal abnormalities, and other medical conditions.

Nurses play a crucial role in assisting patients during the X-ray process. They may explain the procedure to patients, ensure their comfort and safety, and take necessary measures to protect them from unnecessary radiation exposure. This may include placing lead aprons or shields over certain body parts that are not being x-rayed.

Nurses are also responsible for positioning patients correctly to obtain clear and accurate images. They may collaborate with radiology technicians and radiologists to ensure proper imaging techniques and settings are used.

After the X-ray, nurses may assist in the transportation and transfer of the patient back to their room or unit. They may also be involved in the communication of the imaging results to the patient or the healthcare team.

Nursing professionals need to have knowledge of radiation safety procedures and protocols to ensure the well-being of patients and themselves during X-ray procedures. They may also be responsible for documenting the patient's medical history, relevant symptoms, and any precautions taken during the X-ray process in the patient's medical records.

120. Yeast infection

In nursing, a yeast infection refers to an overgrowth of fungus, particularly Candida, in certain areas of the body. The most common type of yeast infection is Candidiasis, which typically affects the skin, mouth, throat, or genital area.

In the context of nursing, yeast infections are often encountered in clinical settings or during patient care. Some examples include:

1. Oral Thrush: This is a yeast infection that affects the mouth and throat, typically seen in patients with weakened immune systems, those on antibiotics, or individuals with poor oral hygiene. Nurses may assess the oral cavity for characteristic white patches or lesions and provide appropriate treatment, such as antifungal medications.

2. Vaginal Candidiasis: Also known as vaginal yeast infection, this occurs due to an overgrowth of Candida in the vaginal area, resulting in symptoms such as itching, burning, and abnormal discharge. Nurses may assess the patient's symptoms, recommend over-the-counter or prescribed antifungal treatment, and provide education on prevention and hygiene.

3. Intertrigo: This refers to a yeast infection that occurs in the skin folds, such as the groin, under the breasts, or between the toes. Nurses may assess the affected area for redness, moisture, and odor, and suggest appropriate treatment options, including antifungal creams or powders, as well as measures to keep the affected area clean and dry.

Nurses play a role in the assessment, identification, and management of yeast infections through patient education, counseling, and administration of prescribed treatments. They also provide support and guidance to patients to prevent future infections by promoting good hygiene practices and addressing any underlying causes or contributing factors.

121. Abdomen

In nursing, the abdomen refers to the region of the body between the chest and the pelvis. It is the area that encompasses various organs and structures, including the stomach, liver, gallbladder, intestines, kidneys, and reproductive organs.

Assessing the abdomen is an important nursing skill that involves performing a comprehensive examination to evaluate the health and functioning of these organs. This may include inspecting the abdomen for any visible abnormalities, such as scars, rashes, or distensions. Nurses may also use palpation to feel for tenderness, masses, or abnormal structures within the abdomen.

In addition to physical assessment, nurses may also be involved in other aspects related to the abdomen in nursing practice. This can include:

1. Gastrointestinal (GI) Care: Nurses play a role in administering medications for GI conditions, educating patients about dietary modifications, and managing symptoms such as nausea, vomiting, or abdominal pain.

2. Wound Care: Nurses may assess and manage surgical incisions or wounds in the abdominal area, ensuring proper wound healing, preventing infection, and providing appropriate dressing changes.

3. Urinary Care: Nurses also monitor and provide care for urinary function and issues related to the lower abdomen, such as urinary catheterization, bladder health, and monitoring urine output.

4. Obstetric Care: Nurses are involved in prenatal and postpartum care, including assessing the pregnant abdomen for fetal growth, monitoring maternal well-being, and providing education on proper positioning and comfort during pregnancy.

Assessing and providing care for the abdomen requires knowledge of anatomy, proper assessment techniques, and understanding of common abdominal conditions and symptoms. Nurses play a critical role in identifying potential issues, monitoring changes, and collaborating with the healthcare team to develop appropriate care plans for patients.

122. Analgesic

In nursing, an analgesic refers to a medication or treatment that is used to relieve or reduce pain. Analgesics work by altering the perception of pain signals in the body and can be administered through various routes, such as oral, topical, intravenous, or intramuscular.

Nurses play a crucial role in the administration and management of analgesic medications as part of pain management interventions. This includes assessing the patient's pain level, monitoring the effectiveness of the analgesic, and evaluating any side effects or adverse reactions.

Nurses may administer analgesics according to the healthcare provider's orders and document the medication administration, dosage, and frequency in the patient's medical records. They may also educate patients and their families about the proper use of analgesics, potential side effects, and the importance of reporting any changes in pain levels.

Additionally, nurses may implement non-pharmacological pain management strategies in conjunction with analgesics. These can include techniques such as heat or cold therapy, massage, distraction techniques, relaxation exercises, or positioning to provide comfort and alleviate pain.

The goal of using analgesics in nursing is to effectively manage pain, improve patient comfort, and enhance the overall well-being of patients. Nurses collaborate with the healthcare team and work with patients to develop individualized pain management plans that consider the type and severity of pain, patient preferences, and any underlying conditions or contraindications for specific analgesic medications.

123. Bronchoscopy

In nursing, bronchoscopy refers to a medical procedure that involves the examination of the airways, specifically the bronchi and lungs. During a bronchoscopy, a thin, flexible instrument called a bronchoscope is inserted through the nose or mouth and down the throat to visualize the airways and collect tissue samples if needed.

Nurses play a critical role in assisting during bronchoscopy procedures and providing pre- and post-operative care. This includes:

1. Pre-procedure: Nurses prepare the patient for the bronchoscopy by obtaining a detailed medical history, explaining the procedure, and obtaining informed consent.

They may also assist in administering medications such as sedatives or local anesthetics to ensure patient comfort during the procedure.

2. Intra-procedure: Nurses are present during the bronchoscopy procedure to assist the physician or respiratory therapist. They help in positioning the patient correctly, ensuring monitoring of vital signs, and providing any necessary suctioning or oxygen supplementation. Nurses also assist with sterile techniques and equipment handling.

3. Post-procedure: After the bronchoscopy, nurses monitor the patient's vital signs, oxygen levels, and any potential complications such as bleeding or difficulty breathing. They assess the patient for any immediate adverse reactions and provide appropriate care. Nurses also provide education and instructions on post-procedure recovery, including activity restrictions, possible side effects, and when to report any complications.

Nurses may also be involved in collecting and labeling any specimens obtained during the bronchoscopy for laboratory analysis, ensuring they are properly handled and transported.

Overall, nurses' roles in bronchoscopy involve pre-procedure preparation, intra-procedure assistance, and post-procedure care to ensure patient safety, comfort, and optimal outcomes.

124. Carbuncle

In nursing, a carbuncle refers to a skin infection that involves a cluster of hair follicles and surrounding tissue. It is a more severe form of a boil, or furuncle, and typically occurs in areas with hair, such as the neck, back, or thighs.

Carbuncles usually develop when bacteria, primarily Staphylococcus aureus, enter the skin through a hair follicle or a small cut or abrasion. The infection causes a painful, swollen, and red lump that may gradually progress to form a cluster of pus-filled boils.

In nursing, the management of a carbuncle involves several key steps:

1. Assessment: Nurses assess the carbuncle's size, appearance, and severity. They may evaluate the patient's vital signs and general health status to determine the extent of the infection and any associated complications.

2. Treatment: Treatment for a carbuncle typically includes the application of warm compresses to help the boil drain, relieve pain, and promote healing. Nurses may educate the patient on correct compress application techniques and advise on the frequency and duration of this treatment.

3. Antibiotics: In some cases, antibiotics may be necessary to treat carbuncles. Nurses may assist in administering oral or intravenous antibiotics as prescribed by the healthcare provider.

4. Incision and Drainage: If the carbuncle does not improve or when an abscess forms, a healthcare provider may need to perform an incision and drainage procedure. Nurses may help prepare the patient for the procedure, assist during the procedure, and provide wound care instructions afterward.

5. Education and Follow-up: Nurses educate patients on proper wound care, including keeping the area clean, applying dressings or ointments as directed, and monitoring for signs of infection. They may also provide information on measures to prevent recurrent carbuncles, such as good hygiene practices and avoiding sharing personal items.

Nurses play an important role in the management of carbuncles by assessing and monitoring the infection, providing appropriate treatment, promoting wound healing, and educating patients on self-care and preventive measures.

125. CHF (congestive heart failure)

In nursing, CHF (congestive heart failure) refers to a chronic condition in which the heart is unable to pump blood effectively, leading to a backlog or congestion of blood in the body. CHF occurs when the heart becomes weakened or damaged, typically due to conditions such as coronary artery disease, high blood pressure, heart valve disorders, or cardiomyopathy.

In nursing, the management of CHF involves several key aspects:

1. Assessment: Nurses assess patients with CHF by monitoring their vital signs, including heart rate, blood pressure, respiratory rate, and oxygen saturation. They also assess signs and symptoms such as shortness of breath, edema (swelling), fatigue, and decreased exercise tolerance. Additionally, nurses may perform physical assessments to identify signs of fluid gain, such as auscultating lung sounds for crackles or assessing dependent edema.

2. Medication Management: Nurses play a crucial role in administering and monitoring medications prescribed to manage CHF. These may include diuretics to reduce fluid overload, ACE inhibitors or angiotensin receptor blockers (ARBs) to improve heart function, beta-blockers to control heart rate, or other medications as determined by the healthcare provider. Nurses educate patients about the purpose, dosage, potential side effects, and importance of medication compliance.

3. Fluid and Sodium Restriction: Nurses provide education and support to patients regarding the importance of adhering to fluid and sodium restrictions. They may provide dietary counseling, assist in developing meal plans, and educate patients on reading food labels and making informed choices to avoid excessive sodium intake.

4. Symptom Management: Nurses assist patients in managing symptoms related to CHF, such as shortness of breath, fatigue, and edema. This may involve teaching

breathing techniques, monitoring weight regularly, and providing strategies for conserving energy and managing fatigue.

5. Patient Education: Nurses play a crucial role in educating patients and their families about CHF, including its causes, signs, symptoms, and management strategies. They provide information on lifestyle modifications, such as maintaining a heart-healthy diet, regular exercise, stress management, and medication adherence. Nurses may also provide education on recognizing and reporting worsening symptoms to seek timely medical attention.

6. Collaboration and Coordination: Nurses collaborate with the healthcare team, including physicians, cardiologists, dieticians, and other specialists, to develop and implement comprehensive care plans for patients with CHF. They communicate patient progress, report changes in symptoms or vital signs, and ensure coordination of care across various healthcare settings.

Through assessment, education, medication management, and coordination of care, nurses play an important role in supporting patients with CHF to manage symptoms, improve quality of life, and prevent exacerbations.

126. CPAP (continuous positive airway pressure)

In nursing, CPAP (continuous positive airway pressure) refers to a medical therapy used to treat individuals with breathing difficulties, particularly those with sleep apnea. It involves the delivery of a continuous flow of air at a prescribed pressure to keep the airways open during sleep and improve breathing.

In the context of nursing, CPAP may involve the following:

1. Assessment: Nurses assess patients for signs and symptoms of sleep apnea, such as excessive daytime sleepiness, loud snoring, observed episodes of breathing cessation during sleep, or morning headaches. They may collaborate with other

healthcare providers, such as sleep specialists, to determine if CPAP therapy is appropriate.

2. Patient Education: Nurses play a key role in educating patients about CPAP therapy. This includes explaining how the equipment works, the benefits of treatment, and the importance of compliance. Nurses guide patients in using and maintaining CPAP devices, including mask fit, cleaning procedures, and troubleshooting common issues.

3. Administration: Nurses may assist in the setup and calibration of CPAP machines, ensuring appropriate pressure settings are programmed for each individual patient. They may demonstrate proper mask fitting techniques and provide guidance on adjusting straps, ensuring a secure and comfortable fit.

4. Monitoring and Follow-up: Nurses monitor patients' adherence to CPAP therapy and assess its effectiveness by evaluating symptom improvement and sleep quality. They provide ongoing support and address any concerns or challenges patients may have with using CPAP. Regular follow-up appointments may be scheduled to evaluate the effectiveness of therapy and make any necessary adjustments.

5. Patient Safety: Nurses ensure patient safety by monitoring for any adverse events related to CPAP therapy, such as skin irritation or pressure sores from mask use. They also educate patients on recognizing and reporting any potential complications, such as air leaks, discomfort, or mask discomfort.

Nurses play an important role in the successful implementation of CPAP therapy by providing education, support, and monitoring to ensure patient adherence and optimal treatment outcomes. They work in collaboration with sleep specialists, respiratory therapists, and other members of the healthcare team to address sleep apnea and improve patients' overall respiratory health.

127. CT scan (computed tomography)

In nursing, a CT scan (computed tomography) refers to a medical imaging procedure that uses a combination of X-rays and computer technology to produce detailed cross-sectional images of the body. CT scans provide clear, high-resolution images that can help diagnose and assess various medical conditions.

In nursing, the management of a patient undergoing a CT scan involves several key aspects:

1. Patient Preparation: Nurses provide pre-procedural care by explaining the CT scan procedure to the patient, ensuring informed consent is obtained, and addressing any questions or concerns. They may also assess the patient's medical history and ensure any necessary precautions or preparations are followed, such as fasting or temporarily discontinuing medications that may interfere with the scan.

2. Contrast Administration: CT scans may involve the use of contrast materials to enhance the visibility of certain structures or organs. Nurses may be responsible for administering contrast agents, either orally, intravenously, or by other routes, while carefully monitoring the patient for any adverse reactions or allergies.

3. Patient Comfort and Safety: Nurses ensure the patient is comfortable during the CT scan, positioning them correctly, and providing any necessary support or assistance. They adhere to radiation safety protocols by shielding and protecting the patient from unnecessary radiation exposure.

4. Education and Support: Nurses play a crucial role in providing education and support to the patient before, during, and after the CT scan. They explain the process, manage any anxieties or fears, and offer reassurance throughout the procedure. After the scan, nurses may inform the patient of any specific post-procedural instructions, such as drinking fluids, resuming normal activities, or monitoring for potential side effects.

5. Post-procedure Care: Nurses monitor the patient post-CT scan, assessing vital signs, any immediate complications, or allergic reactions related to the contrast material. They provide appropriate post-procedure care, including wound care for any biopsy sites or monitoring for any delayed reactions or symptoms.

6. Collaboration and Documentation: Nurses collaborate with the healthcare team, including radiologists and other providers, to ensure prompt interpretation of the CT scan results. Nurses also document the patient's medical history, procedure details, contrast administration, patient response, and any observed complications or reactions in the patient's medical records.

Nurses play a crucial role in ensuring the well-being and safety of patients undergoing CT scans. They provide education, support, and interventions to facilitate a successful procedure, assist with patient comfort, and contribute to the overall effectiveness of the diagnostic imaging process.

128. Cyanosis

In nursing, cyanosis refers to the bluish or purplish discoloration of the skin, mucous membranes, and nails. It is caused by a lack of oxygen in the blood, resulting in inadequate oxygenation of tissues. Cyanosis is a significant clinical sign that may indicate a problem with oxygen delivery to the body tissues.

Nurses play a crucial role in assessing and managing cyanosis in patients. This involves:

1. Assessment: Nurses assess patients for signs of cyanosis, such as a bluish or purplish coloration of the lips, face, nail beds, or extremities. They also consider other associated signs or symptoms, such as shortness of breath, confusion, or altered consciousness. Nurses measure oxygen saturation levels using pulse oximetry, which provides an objective measure of the percentage of oxygen in the blood.

2. Monitoring: Nurses monitor patients with cyanosis closely, paying attention to their respiratory status, heart rate, blood pressure, and overall level of distress. They regularly assess oxygen saturation levels and document any changes or trends.

3. Oxygen Therapy: Nurses may administer oxygen therapy to patients with cyanosis to increase oxygen delivery to the tissues. This can involve using nasal cannulas, face masks, or other oxygen delivery devices, with appropriate flow rates based on the patient's condition and oxygen saturation levels. They monitor the patient's response to oxygen therapy and make adjustments as necessary.

4. Collaboration and Communication: Nurses collaborate with the healthcare team, such as physicians, respiratory therapists, or other specialists, to determine the underlying cause of cyanosis and develop a comprehensive care plan. They communicate changes in the patient's condition and collaborate on interventions aimed at improving oxygenation.

5. Patient and Family Education: Nurses provide education to patients and their families about the significance of cyanosis, potential causes, and the importance of timely intervention. They may educate patients on signs and symptoms to watch for, the proper use of oxygen therapy equipment, and strategies to manage and prevent recurrent cyanosis.

Prompt recognition and management of cyanosis are essential in nursing care. Nurses monitor patients closely, provide interventions to improve oxygenation, and collaborate with the healthcare team to ensure patient safety and optimal outcomes.

129. Dehydration

In nursing, dehydration refers to a condition in which the body does not have enough fluid to function properly. It occurs when the body loses more fluid than it takes in. Dehydration can result from various causes, such as excessive sweating, inadequate fluid intake, vomiting, diarrhea, or certain medical conditions.

In nursing, the assessment and management of dehydration involve several key aspects:

1. Assessment: Nurses assess patients for signs and symptoms of dehydration, which may include increased thirst, dry mouth and lips, fatigue, dizziness, dark-colored urine, decreased urine output, sunken eyes, dry skin, and increased heart rate. They may also consider other factors such as the patient's medical history, recent illness, or medication use.

2. Fluid Balance Monitoring: Nurses monitor the patient's fluid intake and output, measuring urine output and assessing the patient's hydration status. They may also monitor laboratory values such as electrolyte levels, blood urea nitrogen (BUN), and creatinine to evaluate the severity of dehydration and guide treatment.

3. Oral Hydration: Nurses encourage patients to increase their fluid intake through oral hydration methods, offering fluids regularly and assessing the patient's ability to drink and tolerate fluids. They may educate patients on the importance of drinking adequate fluids and provide recommendations for fluid choices.

4. Intravenous (IV) Fluid Therapy: In cases of severe dehydration or when oral fluids are inadequate, nurses may administer intravenous fluids to restore fluid balance. They follow prescribed orders for the type and rate of fluid administration and monitor the patient's response to IV therapy, including vital signs, urine output, and improvements in signs of dehydration.

5. Patient Education: Nurses play a vital role in educating patients and their families about dehydration prevention and management. They provide guidance on the importance of adequate fluid intake, signs of dehydration, and strategies to maintain hydration. Nurses also promote preventive measures, such as drinking water regularly, especially during hot weather or periods of illness.

6. Collaboration and Support: Nurses collaborate with other healthcare professionals, such as physicians, dietitians, or pharmacists, to address the underlying causes of dehydration and develop individualized care plans. They provide support and regular reassessment to ensure the patient's hydration status improves.

Nurses play a critical role in the identification, prevention, and management of dehydration. Their assessments, interventions, and education help maintain fluid balance, improve patient outcomes, and prevent dehydration-related complications.

130. Diabetic

In nursing, "diabetic" refers to a patient who has diabetes. Diabetes is a chronic disease characterized by high levels of blood glucose (sugar) resulting from defects in insulin production, insulin action, or both. Nursing care for diabetic patients involves monitoring blood sugar levels, administering insulin or other medications, educating patients on proper diet and exercise, and managing complications or potential side effects of the disease.

131. Diarrhea

In nursing, "diarrhea" refers to the condition characterized by loose or watery stools, usually occurring with increased frequency. It is a common gastrointestinal symptom that can be caused by various factors such as infections (such as viral or bacterial gastroenteritis), food poisoning, medication side effects, inflammatory bowel diseases, or dietary factors.

Nursing care for patients with diarrhea involves assessing and monitoring the frequency and consistency of stools, monitoring fluid and electrolyte balance, providing hydration through oral rehydration solutions or intravenous fluids if necessary, administering medications to manage symptoms or treat the underlying cause, and educating patients on proper hygiene and dietary modifications to support recovery. Nurses play a crucial role in identifying any complications, such as dehydration or electrolyte imbalances, and implementing appropriate interventions to promote the patient's well-being.

132. Disinfection

In nursing, "disinfection" refers to the process of eliminating or reducing microorganisms on surfaces, equipment, or instruments to a level that is considered safe and free from harmful pathogens. Disinfection is an essential part of infection control practices in healthcare settings.

Nurses are responsible for implementing proper disinfection protocols to prevent the spread of infections. This may involve cleaning and disinfecting patient rooms, equipment, and frequently touched surfaces using appropriate disinfectant solutions. Nurses must follow specific guidelines and protocols provided by infection control experts or their facility's policies to ensure effective disinfection.

Disinfection methods can include using chemical agents, such as disinfectant wipes or sprays, or utilizing automated systems like ultraviolet (UV) light sterilization or hydrogen peroxide vapor systems. Nurses must be knowledgeable about the proper use and application of disinfectants, ensuring that they are used according to manufacturer instructions and in a way that effectively kills or reduces the presence of pathogens.

By implementing rigorous disinfection practices, nurses play a critical role in maintaining a clean and safe healthcare environment, reducing the risk of healthcare-associated infections, and promoting patient safety.

133. Dorsal

In nursing, "dorsal" refers to the back aspect of the body. It is the opposite of ventral, which refers to the front, or anterior, aspect of the body. When referring to anatomical positions or directions, dorsal often indicates the posterior or back side of the body or a specific body part.

For example, in the context of patient assessment, nurses may use the term "dorsal" when documenting the location of a symptom or finding on the back of a patient. This can include describing the presence of rashes, wounds, or pain in specific areas of the back. Nurses also use the term when positioning patients, such as when placing a patient in the dorsal recumbent position, which involves lying flat on the back with the knees flexed.

Understanding anatomical terms like "dorsal" is crucial for effective communication and accurate documentation among healthcare professionals.

134. Dystrophy

In nursing, "dystrophy" refers to a group of genetic disorders that cause muscle weakness and degeneration. Muscular dystrophy is the most well-known type of dystrophy. It is a progressive condition that leads to the weakening and wasting of muscle tissues over time.

Nurses play a role in the care of patients with muscular dystrophy by providing ongoing support, education, and monitoring of symptoms. They may assist in managing the associated physical limitations, such as mobility aids or adaptive equipment, as well as providing emotional support to patients and their families. Nurses also collaborate with other healthcare professionals to develop a comprehensive care plan that addresses the needs and challenges faced by individuals with dystrophy.

135. Echocardiogram

In nursing, an "echocardiogram" refers to a diagnostic test that uses ultrasound technology to produce detailed images of the heart. It provides valuable information about the structure and function of the heart, including the size of the heart chambers, the pumping strength of the heart, and the functioning of the heart valves.

Nurses play an important role in the echocardiogram process. They may assist in preparing patients for the procedure, ensuring that they are comfortable and informed about what to expect. Nurses may also assist the cardiologist or cardiac sonographer during the echocardiogram by positioning the patient, applying gel to the chest area for optimal ultrasound imaging, and reassuring and monitoring the patient throughout the procedure.

After the echocardiogram, nurses may be involved in the interpretation and analysis of the results alongside the healthcare team. They may help educate patients about the findings, answer questions, and provide necessary support or referrals for further evaluation or treatment if abnormalities are detected. Nurses also play a key role in documenting and communicating the echocardiogram findings accurately in the patients' medical records to ensure seamless continuity of care.

136. Edematous

In nursing, "edematous" refers to a condition characterized by the accumulation of excess fluid in the body's tissues, leading to swelling and increased fluid volume. Edema can occur in various parts of the body, including the limbs, abdomen, face, and even the lungs.

Nurses are responsible for assessing and monitoring patients for signs of edema. This may involve examining and palpating the affected areas for swelling, measuring and documenting the size and circumference of the edematous areas, and assessing the skin for changes in texture or color. Nurses also assess for associated symptoms, such as shortness of breath or weight gain, which can indicate more severe or systemic edema.

When managing edema, nurses may implement interventions such as elevating the affected body part, providing compression garments or wraps, promoting adequate rest and mobility, and assisting with fluid management and diuretic therapy as prescribed by the healthcare provider. Nurses also educate patients and their families about strategies to prevent or manage edema, including dietary modifications, medication adherence, exercise, and lifestyle changes.

By monitoring and managing edema, nurses help optimize patients' comfort, mobility, and overall well-being. They collaborate with the interprofessional healthcare team to assess the underlying causes of edema and develop appropriate interventions to address the condition effectively.

137. Electroencephalogram (EEG)

In nursing, an "electroencephalogram" (EEG) refers to a non-invasive diagnostic test that records the electrical activity of the brain. It involves placing electrodes on the scalp to detect and measure the electrical impulses produced by the brain.

Nurses play a critical role in the EEG process. They may help prepare patients for the procedure by explaining what to expect and ensuring they are in a comfortable position. Nurses may also assist in applying the electrodes to the scalp, ensuring proper placement and optimal signal acquisition. During the test, nurses monitor the patient's comfort and safety, as well as their ability to follow instructions given by the EEG technologist.

After the EEG, nurses collaborate with the healthcare team to interpret the results. They may educate patients and their families about the findings, answer questions, and provide support or referrals as needed. Nurses also play a role in documenting and communicating the EEG results accurately in the patient's medical records to facilitate further evaluation or treatment if abnormalities are detected.

Nurses with additional training in neurology or epilepsy may have an expanded role in the management of patients with a suspected or diagnosed neurological condition, including monitoring and managing seizures, administering anti-epileptic medications, and providing education and support to individuals and families affected by epilepsy or other brain disorders.

138. Emesis

Emesis is the medical term for vomiting. In nursing, emesis refers to the act of expelling stomach contents through the mouth due to various reasons such as illness, medications, or anesthesia. Nurses often assess and provide care for patients who are experiencing emesis, which may involve monitoring the frequency and amount of vomiting, offering supportive care, and assessing for potential complications.

In the nursing context, assessing a patient's emesis involves examining the color, consistency, and amount of vomit, as this information can provide important clues about the underlying cause. For example, yellow or green vomit may indicate the presence of bile, while bloody vomit (hematemesis) may suggest gastrointestinal bleeding.

Nurses also assess the frequency of vomiting, as persistent or severe emesis can lead to dehydration, electrolyte imbalances, and other complications. Depending on the patient's condition, nurses may intervene by providing antiemetic medications, intravenous fluids, or other treatments to help manage the vomiting and prevent further complications.

Furthermore, nurses play a crucial role in educating patients about proper nutrition and hydration, especially after episodes of emesis, to ensure that they are properly nourished and hydrated during the recovery process. By closely monitoring and managing emesis, nurses help promote patient comfort and well-being while addressing any underlying issues that may be contributing to the vomiting.

139. Emulsify

In nursing, the term "emulsify" typically refers to the process of breaking down or mixing together two substances that don't naturally mix well, such as oil and water. This can involve using an emulsifying agent to help stabilize the mixture. In healthcare settings, emulsification may be necessary when preparing certain medications or topical treatments that require specific formulations for proper administration or absorption by the body.

140. Febrile

"Febrile" in nursing refers to a condition in which a person has an elevated body temperature, usually as a result of an infection or illness. When a patient is described as febrile, it indicates that they have a fever. Fever is a common symptom that occurs when the body is fighting off an infection or inflammation. In nursing, monitoring a patient's fever is important as it can provide valuable information about their health status and guide treatment decisions. Febrile episodes can vary in severity and duration, with temperatures ranging from slightly elevated to critically high. As a nurse, assessing a febrile patient involves monitoring their temperature regularly, observing for other symptoms such as chills, sweating, and general malaise, and evaluating the potential causes of the fever.

It's crucial for nurses to respond promptly to febrile patients by implementing appropriate interventions to help alleviate their symptoms and address the underlying cause of the fever. Treatment may involve administering antipyretic medications to reduce the fever, maintaining adequate hydration, monitoring vital signs, and closely monitoring the patient's condition for any signs of deterioration. In certain situations, a febrile episode may require further diagnostic tests, such as blood tests or imaging studies, to identify the specific cause of the fever. By closely monitoring and managing febrile patients, nurses play a vital role in supporting their recovery and ensuring optimal outcomes.

141. Flatus

To refer to the passing of gas from the digestive system through the rectum. It is a normal bodily function that can sometimes be a source of discomfort or embarrassment for patients. Nurses may assess and address issues related to flatus as part of their care for patients. On the patient's condition and comfort level. Nurses may educate patients on dietary changes that could help reduce excessive gas production or offer medications to alleviate discomfort associated with flatus. Assessing the frequency and characteristics of flatus can also provide valuable information about a patient's digestive health and overall well-being.

Additionally, nurses may use their expertise to differentiate between normal flatus and symptoms that could indicate underlying digestive problems, such as excessive bloating, foul-smelling gas, or changes in bowel habits. By addressing issues related to flatus in a sensitive and professional manner, nurses play a crucial role in promoting patient comfort and digestive health.

142. Gait

Gait in nursing refers to the pattern of walking or the manner in which a person walks. Nurses may assess a patient's gait as part of a physical examination to evaluate their balance, coordination, and overall mobility. Changes in gait can sometimes indicate underlying health issues or be a result of certain medical conditions, injuries, or neurological impairments. Some of the key aspects that nurses look for when assessing a patient's gait include the person's posture, balance, stride length, step width, arm swing, and coordination. Abnormalities in any of these aspects may suggest a potential issue that needs further evaluation or intervention.

Assessing gait is important in nursing care because it can provide valuable information about a patient's overall functional status and help in formulating an appropriate care plan. For example, a nurse may observe changes in gait that could be indicative of an increased fall risk, muscle weakness, joint problems, or neurological conditions.

Nurses may also collaborate with other healthcare professionals, such as physical therapists or physicians, to further evaluate and address any gait abnormalities identified during assessment. Developing interventions and strategies to improve gait can help enhance a patient's mobility, independence, and overall quality of life.

Overall, gait assessment is an essential aspect of nursing care that allows healthcare providers to gather important information about a patient's physical well-being and functional abilities, ultimately guiding appropriate care and treatment decisions.

143. Hematocrit

Hematocrit in nursing refers to the proportion of red blood cells in the blood. It is an important measurement that helps in evaluating the blood's ability to carry oxygen and in diagnosing various medical conditions, such as anemia or polycythemia. The hematocrit level is expressed as a percentage of the total volume of blood that is made up of red blood cells. Hematocrit levels are commonly measured through a simple blood test called a hematocrit test. The normal range of hematocrit can vary based on factors like age, sex, and altitude. Low hematocrit levels may indicate conditions such as anemia, blood loss, malnutrition, or bone marrow disorders. On the other hand, high hematocrit levels may be a sign of conditions like dehydration, polycythemia vera, or lung diseases.

In nursing practice, monitoring hematocrit levels is essential for assessing a patient's overall health status, response to treatment, and progression of certain diseases. Nurses play a vital role in educating patients about the significance of hematocrit levels, potential causes of abnormal results, and the importance of follow-up care. Additionally, nurses may administer treatments or interventions based on hematocrit levels to ensure optimal patient outcomes.

144. Hemoglobin

Hemoglobin in nursing refers to a protein found in red blood cells that is responsible for carrying oxygen throughout the body. It plays a crucial role in maintaining proper oxygen levels in the blood, which is essential for the body's functioning. Nurses often monitor hemoglobin levels in patients to assess their overall health and to help diagnose conditions such as anemia or other blood disorders. Hemoglobin levels can give important insights into a person's overall well-being and help guide treatment decisions in nursing care.

Hemoglobin is composed of heme, which contains iron, allowing it to bind with oxygen molecules in the lungs and transport them to tissues and organs throughout the body. Monitoring hemoglobin levels is a common practice in nursing, as it can provide important information about a patient's oxygen-carrying capacity and overall health status. Low hemoglobin levels, known as anemia, can lead to symptoms such as fatigue, weakness, and shortness of breath, while high levels may indicate dehydration, polycythemia, or other underlying health conditions.

Nurses may perform hemoglobin tests as part of routine blood work, especially in settings such as hospitals, clinics, and primary care offices. Understanding a patient's hemoglobin level can help nurses and other healthcare providers make informed decisions about treatment plans, monitor the effectiveness of interventions, and evaluate the need for further testing or specialized care. Overall, hemoglobin plays a critical role in maintaining the body's oxygen balance, and nurses play a key role in assessing and managing hemoglobin levels to support optimal patient outcomes.

145. Hemorrhoid

Hemorrhoids in nursing refer to swollen or inflamed veins in the rectum and anus that can cause discomfort, pain, itching, and sometimes bleeding. Nurses may encounter patients who are experiencing hemorrhoids and may need to provide education, care, and support for managing this condition. Treatment options for hemorrhoids may include lifestyle changes, topical medications, or surgical interventions, depending on the severity of the symptoms. Hemorrhoids, also known as piles, can be internal or external. Internal hemorrhoids develop inside the rectum, while external hemorrhoids form under the skin around the anal opening. Contributing factors to hemorrhoids can include straining during bowel movements, chronic constipation or diarrhea, pregnancy, obesity, and a sedentary lifestyle.

In nursing care, management of hemorrhoids involves assessing the patient's symptoms, providing education on proper bowel habits and dietary changes, recommending over-the-counter treatments like topical creams or suppositories, and advising on sitz baths for relief. Nurses may also collaborate with healthcare providers to determine if further interventions such as banding, sclerotherapy, or surgery are needed for severe cases.

Supporting patients with hemorrhoids includes addressing their discomfort, ensuring proper hygiene, monitoring for complications such as excessive bleeding or thrombosis, and promoting strategies to prevent recurrence. Nurses play a vital role in helping patients manage hemorrhoids effectively and improve their quality of life.

146. Hygiene

Hygiene in nursing pertains to the practices and measures taken by healthcare professionals to maintain cleanliness, prevent infections, and promote the overall health and well-being of patients. Proper hygiene practices in nursing include handwashing, wound care, sterilization of equipment, patient bathing, oral care, and environmental cleanliness. Good hygiene is essential in preventing the spread of infections and ensuring optimal patient care. Good hygiene practices in nursing also involve the maintenance of a clean and safe healthcare environment. This includes regular cleaning and disinfection of patient rooms, equipment, and common areas to prevent the spread of harmful bacteria and viruses. Nurses are also responsible for ensuring that patients receive proper personal hygiene care, such as bathing, grooming, and changing soiled bedding or clothing.

In addition, hygiene in nursing involves practicing proper infection control techniques, such as wearing personal protective equipment (PPE) like gloves, masks, and gowns when necessary, to protect both the healthcare provider and the patient from the transmission of infectious diseases. Nurses are also trained to follow strict protocols for handling and disposing of contaminated materials to prevent the spread of infections.

Overall, maintaining high standards of hygiene is crucial in nursing to prevent healthcare-associated infections, promote patient safety, and support the overall health and well-being of patients under their care.

147. Immobilize

In nursing, "immobilize" means to prevent movement of a part of the body, such as a limb or a joint, often using splints, straps, or braces. This may be done to stabilize fractures, prevent further injury, or support healing. Immobilization can also be used in cases of muscle strains, sprains, or conditions that require restricted movement for proper recovery

148. Impaired

Impaired in nursing typically refers to a nurse's ability to safely and effectively perform their job due to physical, mental, or emotional issues such as substance abuse, mental health conditions, or physical limitations. When a nurse is considered impaired, it can pose risks to patient safety and necessitate interventions such as treatment, monitoring, or even suspension of their nursing license until they are deemed fit to practice again.

149. Infarct

An infarct in nursing refers to an area of tissue that has died due to a lack of blood supply. This occurs when blood flow to a specific part of the body is blocked, leading to tissue death. Infarcts can occur in various organs of the body, such as the heart, brain, or other tissues, and can have serious implications depending on the location and extent of the damage. Nursing care for patients with infarcts typically involves monitoring vital signs, administering medications, and providing support to help manage symptoms and facilitate recovery.

150. Ingest

"Ingest" in nursing refers to the process of taking in food, fluids, or medications by mouth. It is an essential part of a patient's care to ensure proper nutrition, hydration, and administration of prescribed medications. Nurses often monitor and assess a patient's ability to ingest these substances as part of their overall care plan.

151. Intake

Intake in nursing refers to the process of recording and monitoring a patient's fluid and food intake. This may include tracking the amount of water consumed, as well as monitoring the types and quantities of food eaten by the patient. Nurses often record intake measurements to ensure that patients are receiving appropriate nutrition and hydration during their hospital stay or treatment. Tracking intake is important for monitoring the patient's overall health and well-being.

152. Ischemia

I'd be happy to help! Ischemia in nursing refers to a condition where there is decreased blood flow and oxygen supply to a certain part of the body, usually due to a blockage in a blood vessel. This can lead to tissue damage or cell death if not treated promptly. In nursing, it is important to recognize the signs and symptoms of ischemia, such as pain, numbness, or weakness in the affected area, in order to provide appropriate care and prevent further complications. Nurses may also be involved in assessing and monitoring patients at risk for ischemia, as well as implementing interventions to improve blood flow and oxygenation to the affected tissues.

Ischemia can occur in various parts of the body, such as the heart (causing a heart attack), brain (leading to a stroke), or limbs (resulting in peripheral arterial disease). In nursing practice, it is crucial to assess patients for risk factors that can contribute to ischemia, such as obesity, smoking, diabetes, hypertension, and high cholesterol. Nurses play a key role in educating patients about lifestyle modifications and medication adherence to help prevent ischemic events.

During patient care, nurses need to closely monitor individuals with known or suspected ischemia, assessing vital signs, performing neurovascular checks, and observing for changes in pain levels or tissue color and temperature. Prompt recognition of ischemic symptoms is essential to ensure rapid intervention and minimize tissue damage. Nurses may also collaborate with other healthcare professionals, such as physicians and physical therapists, to develop a comprehensive care plan for patients with ischemia.

In addition, nurses often provide emotional support and education to patients and their families regarding the impact of ischemia on their health and well-being. By taking a holistic approach to care, nurses can help patients better manage their condition, improve their quality of life, and reduce the risk of recurrent ischemic events.

153. Laryngitis

Laryngitis is the inflammation of the larynx (voice box) due to overuse, irritation, or infection. In nursing, it refers to the condition where a person experiences hoarseness, loss of voice, or difficulty speaking due to inflammation of the vocal cords. Nursing care for laryngitis typically involves voice rest, hydration, steam inhalation, and sometimes medications to reduce inflammation or manage symptoms. Nursing care for laryngitis also involves educating the patient on vocal hygiene practices to prevent further irritation of the vocal cords. This may include advising the patient to avoid shouting, speaking in noisy environments, smoking, and excessive throat clearing. Additionally, recommending warm beverages, such as herbal teas with honey, can help soothe the throat and alleviate discomfort.

In some cases, a healthcare provider may recommend voice therapy to help the patient learn how to speak or sing without straining the vocal cords. If laryngitis is caused by a bacterial infection, antibiotics may be prescribed. However, if it is due to a viral infection, supportive care such as rest, hydration, and symptom management is usually recommended.

Overall, nursing care for laryngitis focuses on providing comfort, promoting vocal rest and healing, and preventing further complications. Patients with laryngitis are encouraged to follow their healthcare provider's recommendations and seek medical attention if their symptoms worsen or do not improve with home care measures.

154. Lumbar puncture

A lumbar puncture, also known as a spinal tap, is a medical procedure performed to collect and analyze cerebrospinal fluid (CSF) from the space around the spinal cord in the lower back. In nursing, nurses may assist healthcare providers in preparing the patient for the procedure, positioning them correctly, providing support and comfort during the procedure, and monitoring the patient for any complications afterwards. Nurses may also be involved in post-procedure care and education for patients who have undergone a lumbar puncture.

155. Lymph nodes

Lymph nodes are small, bean-shaped structures found throughout the body that play a crucial role in the immune system. In nursing, understanding the location and function of lymph nodes is important for assessing and monitoring a patient's health. Lymph nodes help filter and trap infectious agents, abnormal cells, and other foreign substances, allowing the immune system to mount a response to combat infections and diseases. Nursing assessments may include checking for enlarged or tender lymph nodes, which can indicate inflammation or an underlying health issue that requires further evaluation.

156. Malignancy

Malignancy in the context of nursing refers to the presence of cancerous cells or tumors in the body. Nurses who encounter patients with malignancies often play a crucial role in their care by providing necessary monitoring, support, and education throughout the treatment process. They may also assist in managing symptoms and side effects of cancer therapies to help improve the patient's quality of life.

Malignancy in nursing encompasses a range of conditions involving the growth and spread of cancer cells within the body. Nurses caring for patients with malignancies are responsible for assessing their physical and emotional needs, providing education on the disease and treatment options, and offering support throughout the journey. They collaborate with the healthcare team to develop and implement individualized care plans, monitor patients for complications, administer treatments as prescribed, and advocate for their well-being.

Nurses working with cancer patients often assist in managing side effects such as pain, nausea, fatigue, and emotional distress. They play a vital role in helping patients cope with the challenges of a cancer diagnosis, treatment, and survivorship. Additionally, nurses in oncology settings may provide important education on preventive measures, symptom recognition, and lifestyle changes to promote overall health and well-being.

Overall, nurses caring for patients with malignancies demonstrate compassion, empathy, and expertise in delivering comprehensive care that addresses the physical, emotional, and psychological aspects of cancer treatment. Their dedication and commitment contribute significantly to supporting patients and their families through the complexities of facing and overcoming cancer.

157. Meningitis

Meningitis is a serious condition characterized by inflammation of the protective membranes covering the brain and spinal cord. In nursing, understanding meningitis is crucial as it helps nurses recognize the signs and symptoms, provide appropriate care, and educate patients and families about the condition. Nurses play a critical role in the assessment, treatment, and management of patients with meningitis to ensure optimal outcomes and prevent complications.

158. Micturition

Micturition in nursing refers to the process of urination or the act of emptying the bladder. It involves the coordination of various muscles and nerves to release urine from the body. Nursing professionals often assess and monitor micturition to ensure proper urinary function and address any issues related to urination.

159. Myalgia

Myalgia in nursing refers to muscle pain or aching, which can be caused by various factors such as overuse, injury, infection, or certain medical conditions. Nursing assessment and care for patients with myalgia may involve identifying the underlying cause of the muscle pain, providing pain relief measures, and developing a treatment plan to address the discomfort and promote healing.

Nurses play a crucial role in assessing and managing myalgia in patients. When a patient presents with muscle pain, nurses will conduct a thorough assessment to determine the location, intensity, and duration of the pain. It is important for nurses to gather information about the patient's medical history, recent activities, and any other symptoms that may be present.

Once the assessment is complete, nurses may implement various interventions to help alleviate the muscle pain. This can include administering pain medication, applying heat or cold therapy, performing gentle massages, or recommending rest and appropriate physical activity modifications.

In addition to managing the symptoms of myalgia, nurses also work to educate patients about self-care strategies to prevent future episodes of muscle pain. This may involve teaching patients about proper body mechanics, ergonomics, stretching exercises, and relaxation techniques that can help reduce muscle tension and prevent injury.

Overall, by providing comprehensive care and support to patients with myalgia, nurses can help improve the individual's quality of life and promote a faster recovery from muscle pain.

160. Nasal cannula

A nasal cannula is a medical device used in the field of nursing and healthcare to deliver supplemental oxygen to patients in need. It consists of a lightweight plastic tube that splits into two prongs, which are inserted into the patient's nostrils. The other end of the tubing is connected to an oxygen source, allowing the patient to receive a controlled flow of oxygen to help with breathing. Nasal cannulas are commonly used for patients who require low to moderate levels of supplemental oxygen.

161. Necrosis

Necrosis in nursing refers to the death of cells or tissues in the body due to disease, injury, or lack of blood flow. It is a serious condition that can lead to further complications if not addressed promptly. Nurses play a crucial role in assessing and managing necrosis in patients to prevent its progression and promote healing.

162. Neuropathy

Neuropathy in nursing refers to a condition where there is damage to the nerves, leading to symptoms such as numbness, tingling, muscle weakness, and pain. It can be caused by various factors like diabetes, infections, trauma, or exposure to toxins. Nurses play a vital role in assessing and managing patients with neuropathy, providing education, support, and treatments to help alleviate symptoms and improve quality of life.

163. Nystagmus

Nystagmus is a term used in nursing and medicine to describe a condition characterized by involuntary, repetitive, and uncontrolled eye movements. These movements can be side-to-side (horizontal nystagmus), up and down (vertical nystagmus), or rotary. Nystagmus can be indicative of various underlying health conditions, such as neurological disorders, vestibular (inner ear) issues, or drug toxicity. It is important for nursing professionals to assess and understand nystagmus in their patients as it can provide valuable diagnostic insight.

164. Ocular

Ocular nursing refers to anything related to the eyes or vision. Nurses may assess ocular health, document findings related to the eyes, administer eye medications, or provide education on eye care and safety. The term "ocular" is used to describe conditions, assessments, treatments, and interventions pertaining to the eyes within the nursing field.

165. Orthostatic

Orthostatic in nursing refers to a condition known as orthostatic hypotension, which occurs when a person's blood pressure drops significantly when they move from lying down to standing up. This can result in symptoms such as dizziness, lightheadedness, and fainting. Nurses often monitor for orthostatic hypotension in patients, especially those at risk, to prevent falls and other complications.

166. Otitis

Otitis is a medical term used to describe inflammation or infection of the ear. It can refer to different types of ear infections such as otitis externa (infection of the outer ear canal), otitis media (infection of the middle ear), or otitis interna (infection of the inner ear). In nursing, otitis would involve assessing and managing ear infections, providing appropriate care and treatment, and educating patients about preventive measures and medication management for ear health.

167. Palliative

Palliative care in nursing refers to the specialized medical care provided to patients with serious illnesses to improve their quality of life. The focus of palliative care is on managing pain and other distressing symptoms, providing emotional support, and addressing the overall well-being of the patient and their family. It aims to enhance comfort and promote dignity for patients with life-limiting illnesses, rather than focusing on curative treatment. Palliative care is often provided alongside other medical treatments to help patients cope with the physical, emotional, and spiritual challenges that come with their illness.

168. Paresthesia

Paresthesia in nursing refers to the sensation of numbness, tingling or prickling in the skin, often described as a "pins and needles" feeling. This sensation can occur due to various reasons such as nerve damage, pressure on nerves, poor circulation, or other medical conditions. Nurses need to be aware of paresthesia as it can be a symptom of underlying health issues or complications in patients, and they should monitor and report any instances of paresthesia to the healthcare team for further evaluation and treatment.

169. Pathogen

A pathogen in nursing refers to a microorganism, such as a bacterium, virus, fungus, or parasite, that can cause disease in humans. Nursing professionals need to be aware of various pathogens and how they can be transmitted in order to effectively prevent and control infections in healthcare settings. Understanding pathogens is crucial for maintaining a safe and healthy environment for both patients and healthcare workers.

170. Peritoneal

Peritoneal in nursing refers to the peritoneum, which is the serous membrane that lines the abdominal cavity and covers the abdominal organs. Peritoneal in nursing may be associated with procedures like peritoneal dialysis, which involves using the peritoneum as a membrane for exchanging fluids and removing waste products from the body.

171. Pharyngitis

Pharyngitis in nursing refers to inflammation of the pharynx, which is the part of the throat behind the mouth and nasal cavity. Pharyngitis can be caused by various factors such as viral or bacterial infections, irritants, or allergies. Typical symptoms of pharyngitis include sore throat, difficulty swallowing, and swollen lymph nodes. Nursing care for pharyngitis may involve providing comfort measures, administering medications as prescribed, encouraging adequate hydration, and educating patients on self-care practices.

172. Pleura

The pleura is a thin membrane that lines the chest cavity and covers the lungs. It plays a crucial role in the respiratory system by creating a fluid-filled space that allows the lungs to expand and contract efficiently during breathing. Nurses commonly encounter issues related to the pleura in various conditions such as pleurisy, pleural effusion, or pneumothorax. Understanding the anatomy and function of the pleura is important for nurses when assessing and caring for patients with respiratory problems.

173. Posterior

The term "posterior" in nursing is commonly used to refer to the back side of the body or a specific part of the body that is located at the rear. For example, when a nurse mentions assessing the patient's posterior, they are likely referring to examining the back side of the patient's body for any signs of injury, skin issues, or other abnormalities. It is important for nurses to conduct thorough assessments of both the anterior (front) and posterior (back) parts of the body to ensure comprehensive care for their patients.

174. Prone

In nursing, the term "prone" refers to a body position in which a patient lies on their stomach with their head turned to one side. This position may be used for certain medical procedures or to assist with managing conditions such as acute respiratory distress syndrome (ARDS) or to aid in the drainage of respiratory secretions. Healthcare providers may place patients in the prone position to improve oxygenation or ventilation in some cases.

175. Protocol

A protocol in nursing is a set of guidelines or instructions that delineate the procedures and best practices for specific nursing interventions or treatments. These protocols provide standardized procedures to ensure consistent and quality care for patients. Nurses follow these protocols to deliver evidence-based care and uphold patient safety and well-being.

176. Pruritus

Pruritus in nursing refers to the medical term for itching, which is a common symptom reported by patients. It can result from various conditions such as dry skin, allergies, skin infections, insect bites, medications, and certain systemic diseases. Nursing assessment and management of pruritus are crucial to help relieve discomfort and identify underlying causes that may require further treatment.

177. PTP (prior to procedure)

It means "before operation." During this time, you will meet with one of your doctors. This may be your surgeon or primary care doctor: This checkup usually needs to be done within the month before surgery. This gives your doctors time to treat any medical problems you may have before your surgery.

178. Pulmonary embolism

A pulmonary embolism in nursing refers to a blockage in one of the pulmonary arteries in the lungs, usually caused by a blood clot that travels to the lungs from another part of the body, such as the legs. This condition can be life-threatening and requires immediate medical attention. Nurses play a crucial role in recognizing the signs and symptoms of pulmonary embolism, initiating appropriate interventions, and providing care to patients with this condition.

179. Renal

The term "renal" in nursing typically refers to aspects related to the kidneys. Nurses often encounter the term "renal" when discussing conditions, assessments, treatments, or procedures concerning the kidneys. Patients with renal issues may require specialized care and monitoring to ensure their kidney function is properly managed.

180. Resuscitation

Resuscitation in nursing refers to the process of reviving or restoring a patient's vital functions that have ceased or are at risk of cessation. This can involve techniques such as cardiopulmonary resuscitation (CPR), defibrillation, airway management, and the administration of medications to stabilize the patient. Nurses play a crucial role in resuscitation efforts, particularly in settings such as hospitals, emergency rooms, and intensive care units.

181. Rhinorrhea

Rhinorrhea in nursing refers to the medical term for a runny nose. In nursing, it may be an important symptom to monitor and manage, especially in patients with respiratory conditions or infections. Nurses may assess the color, consistency, and frequency of the nasal discharge to help diagnose and treat underlying conditions.

182. Seizure

A seizure in nursing refers to a sudden, uncontrolled electrical disturbance in the brain that can cause changes in behavior, movements, or consciousness. During a seizure, a person may experience muscle spasms, convulsions, loss of consciousness, or other symptoms. Nurses are trained to recognize seizures, provide immediate care during a seizure to ensure the person's safety, and assist in managing seizures with appropriate medications and interventions.

183. Sigmoidoscopy

A sigmoidoscopy is a medical procedure commonly used by healthcare professionals, including nurses, to examine the inside of the lower part of the large intestine (sigmoid colon) and rectum. During a sigmoidoscopy, a flexible, narrow tube with a camera on the end, called a sigmoidoscope, is inserted through the rectum to visualize and diagnose conditions such as hemorrhoids, inflammation, polyps, or cancer in the sigmoid colon and rectum. Nurses may assist in preparing patients for the procedure, providing education and support, as well as assisting the healthcare provider during the sigmoidoscopy.

184. Sinusitis

Sinusitis in nursing refers to the inflammation or swelling of the tissue lining the sinuses. Sinuses are air-filled spaces in the skull around the nose and eyes. When these spaces become blocked and filled with fluid, it can lead to an infection. Symptoms of sinusitis can include facial pain or pressure, nasal congestion, headache, and thick nasal discharge. Nursing care for patients with sinusitis may involve assessing and managing their symptoms, providing education on medication use and home care, and monitoring for any complications.

185. Sputum

Sputum in nursing refers to the mucus that is expelled from the respiratory tract, typically through coughing. Nurses often observe and assess sputum as part of their patient care to gather information about respiratory health. Changes in the color, consistency, and amount of sputum can provide valuable insights into various respiratory conditions.

186. Sterilization

Sterilization in nursing refers to the process of destroying all microorganisms, including bacteria, viruses, fungi, and spores, to prevent the transmission of infections. In healthcare settings, sterilization is essential to ensure that medical instruments, equipment, and surfaces are free from harmful microorganisms that could potentially cause infections in patients. There are different methods of sterilization, such as autoclaving, chemical sterilization, and radiation sterilization, that are used depending on the specific healthcare setting and the items being sterilized. Sterilization is a critical component of infection control practices in nursing and healthcare to maintain patient safety.

187. Suppository

A suppository in nursing is a medication that is typically cone-shaped and designed to be inserted into a bodily orifice, such as the rectum, vagina, or urethra. It is used for the controlled and localized administration of medication.

188. Syncope

Syncope in nursing refers to a temporary loss of consciousness caused by a drop in blood flow to the brain. It is also known as fainting or passing out. Syncope can be caused by various factors such as dehydration, low blood sugar, heart problems, or sudden changes in posture. Nursing professionals need to assess patients who experience syncope to determine the underlying cause and provide appropriate care.

189. Tachycardia

In nursing, tachycardia refers to a condition where the heart beats faster than normal. It is typically defined as a heart rate greater than 100 beats per minute in adults. Tachycardia can be caused by various factors such as stress, exertion, illness, or certain medical conditions. Nursing professionals monitor and assess patients with tachycardia to determine the underlying cause and provide appropriate care and treatment.

190. Thrombosis

Thrombosis in nursing refers to the formation of a blood clot within a blood vessel that obstructs blood flow. Nurses play a crucial role in assessing, preventing, and managing thrombosis in patients by implementing preventive measures, monitoring for signs and symptoms, and providing appropriate interventions such as administering anticoagulants or arranging for imaging studies to confirm the presence of a clot. Thrombosis can lead to serious complications if not promptly diagnosed and treated, so early recognition and intervention are essential in nursing care.

191. Tidal volume

Tidal volume in nursing refers to the amount of air that enters and leaves the lungs during normal breathing. It represents the volume of air moved into and out of the lungs with each breath. Tidal volume is an important parameter to monitor in patients, especially those with respiratory conditions, as it can indicate how effectively the lungs are functioning. Changes in tidal volume can provide valuable information about a patient's respiratory status and help healthcare providers make treatment decisions.

192. Topical

"Topical" in nursing typically refers to medications or treatments that are applied directly to a specific area of the body, usually the skin or mucous membranes. Topical medications can include creams, ointments, lotions, and patches that are absorbed through the skin to treat localized conditions such as skin infections, rashes, wounds, or pain. Topical treatments are often used for their specific and targeted effects without affecting the rest of the body systemically.

193. Tourniquet

A tourniquet in nursing is a constricting or compressing device used to control bleeding by temporarily stopping the flow of blood through a blood vessel. It is often used during medical procedures, such as drawing blood or starting an intravenous line, to make veins more visible and accessible. Tourniquets should be applied carefully and for a limited time to avoid causing damage to the underlying tissues.

194. Toxin

In nursing, the term "toxin" is used to refer to a poisonous substance that is produced within living cells or organisms and can cause harm when introduced into the body. Toxins can come from a variety of sources such as bacteria, fungi, plants, and animals. Nurses need to be knowledgeable about the different types of toxins, their effects on the body, and the appropriate treatments for toxin exposure or poisoning.

195. Tube feeding

Tube feeding in nursing refers to the administration of nutrients, fluids, or medications through a tube directly into the gastrointestinal tract. This method is used when a patient is unable to consume food orally or when they require additional nutritional support. Tube feeding can be delivered through different types of tubes, such as nasogastric tubes, gastrostomy tubes, or jejunostomy tubes, depending on the patient's condition and needs. Nursing care for patients receiving tube feeding includes monitoring the tube placement, managing the feeding schedule and rate, assessing for complications, and providing patient education and support.

196. Tumor

In nursing, a tumor refers to an abnormal growth of tissue that can be benign (non-cancerous) or malignant (cancerous). Nurses play a crucial role in caring for patients with tumors by monitoring their condition, administering treatments, providing education, and offering support to help manage symptoms and improve quality of life.

197. Ultrasonography

Ultrasonography in nursing refers to the use of ultrasound technology by nurses to visualize and assess internal structures of the body for diagnostic purposes. Nurses may perform or assist in ultrasound procedures to help diagnose medical conditions, monitor fetal development during pregnancy, or guide interventions such as needle placements or catheter insertions. Ultrasonography is a non-invasive imaging technique that uses high-frequency sound waves to create images of organs, tissues, and blood vessels in real-time. In nursing practice, ultrasonography can provide valuable information to support clinical decision-making and patient care.

198. Urethra

The urethra is a tube that carries urine from the bladder to the outside of the body. In nursing, understanding the anatomy and function of the urethra is important for assessing and managing various urinary conditions and issues. Nurses may need to assist patients with catheter insertion, perform urinary catheter care, and educate patients on maintaining good urinary health. Understanding the role of the urethra is crucial for providing high-quality nursing care to patients with urinary system concerns.

199. Urology

Urology in nursing refers to the specialized branch of nursing that focuses on the care of patients with urinary system disorders and conditions. Urology nurses are trained to provide care for patients with various urological issues, such as urinary tract infections, kidney stones, incontinence, prostate disorders, and urinary tract cancers. They work closely with urologists to assess patients, develop treatment plans, provide patient education, and offer support throughout the patient's journey to recovery. Urology nurses play a crucial role in helping patients manage their urological conditions and maintain optimal urological health.

200. Varicella

"Varicella" in nursing refers to the medical term for chickenpox, a common and highly contagious viral infection characterized by an itchy rash of red spots. Nurses may come across cases of varicella in patients, especially in pediatric populations.

Nurses play a crucial role in managing varicella cases by providing supportive care, monitoring for complications, and educating patients and families about the infection. They may also administer medications to alleviate itching and discomfort, as well as ensure infection control measures to prevent the spread of the virus to others. Understanding the signs and symptoms of varicella and knowing how to care for patients with this condition are important aspects of nursing practice.

201. Void

In nursing, "void" refers to the act of urination, specifically when a patient urinates. Nurses often use this term when documenting and communicating information about a patient's urinary output and bladder function. Voiding is an essential physiological function that allows the body to eliminate waste products through the urinary system. In nursing practice, monitoring a patient's voiding patterns and volume is crucial for assessing their overall health and hydration status. Nurses may keep track of the frequency, amount, color, and odor of a patient's urine output to detect any abnormalities or changes that could indicate health issues. Proper documentation of voiding patterns helps healthcare providers make informed decisions about a patient's care and treatment plan. In situations where a patient is unable to void independently, nurses may need to assist with interventions such as catheterization to ensure proper bladder emptying and prevent urinary retention.

202. Vomiting

Vomiting in nursing refers to the involuntary expulsion of stomach contents through the mouth and sometimes through the nose. In nursing, it is important to monitor and assess patients who are vomiting for various reasons, such as infections, gastrointestinal issues, side effects of medications, or as a symptom of an underlying condition. Nurses may provide care and support to patients who are experiencing vomiting, including assessing hydration status, providing antiemetic medications, monitoring for signs of complications, and addressing any underlying causes.

203. Waist circumference

Waist circumference in nursing refers to a measurement taken around the waist at a specific point, usually at the level of the navel. It is a clinical measurement used to assess abdominal obesity and determine the risk of certain health conditions such as heart disease, diabetes, and metabolic syndrome. Nurses often measure waist circumference as part of a comprehensive health assessment to evaluate a patient's overall health status and risk factors.

Waist circumference measurement is a valuable tool in healthcare because it provides information about the distribution of body fat, particularly abdominal fat. Excess fat around the waist can be a sign of visceral fat accumulation, which is linked to an increased risk of various health problems. In nursing practice, waist circumference measurement is often carried out along with other assessments such as body mass index (BMI) calculation and overall health history to get a more comprehensive picture of a patient's health status.

Nurses use standardized guidelines to interpret waist circumference measurements based on gender and ethnicity-specific cutoff points. These guidelines help identify individuals who may be at a higher risk of developing obesity-related health conditions. By regularly monitoring changes in waist circumference over time, healthcare providers can track the effectiveness of interventions such as diet modifications, exercise programs, and weight management strategies in reducing abdominal fat and improving overall health outcomes.

204. Wheezing

"Wheezing" in nursing refers to a high-pitched whistling sound that occurs when air flows through narrowed or constricted airways in the lungs. It is commonly associated with conditions such as asthma, bronchitis, or other respiratory issues. Wheezing can be a sign of airway obstruction and should be assessed by a healthcare provider to determine the underlying cause and appropriate treatment.

The presence of wheezing in a patient can indicate a variety of respiratory conditions, ranging from mild to severe. Asthma, a chronic inflammatory condition that affects the airways, is a common cause of wheezing. During an asthma attack, the airways become inflamed and constricted, leading to difficulty breathing and the characteristic wheezing sound.

Other conditions that can cause wheezing include bronchitis, chronic obstructive pulmonary disease (COPD), pneumonia, or even allergic reactions. Wheezing can also occur due to physical obstructions in the airways, such as a foreign object or a tumor.

In a clinical setting, nurses play a crucial role in assessing patients with wheezing, monitoring their respiratory status, and providing appropriate care. It is essential for nurses to promptly recognize wheezing, assess the patient's overall condition, and collaborate with other healthcare team members to determine the underlying cause and plan effective treatment interventions.

Depending on the cause of wheezing, treatment may involve medications such as bronchodilators, corticosteroids, or antibiotics, as well as oxygen therapy or other supportive measures. Education and counseling on proper inhaler use, environmental triggers, and self-management techniques are also important aspects of nursing care for patients with wheezing.

Overall, wheezing in nursing practice requires thorough assessment, monitoring, and collaborative care to ensure the best possible outcomes for patients with respiratory issues.

205. Abscess

An abscess in nursing refers to a localized collection of pus that forms within tissues of the body as a result of infection. Abscesses can occur in various parts of the body and are typically accompanied by symptoms such as swelling, redness, warmth, and pain. In nursing, managing abscesses involves assessing the size and location of the abscess, providing proper wound care, administering antibiotics if necessary, and ensuring proper drainage and healing.

nursing care for abscesses may involve assessing the patient's overall health status, monitoring for signs of systemic infection, and implementing appropriate treatment protocols. This might include incision and drainage procedures to release the pus and promote healing, as well as dressing changes and wound care to prevent further infection. Nurses also play a crucial role in educating patients about proper wound care, hygiene practices, and the importance of completing any prescribed antibiotic therapy. Additionally, they may collaborate with other healthcare team members, such as physicians and wound care specialists, to ensure optimal management of the abscess and promote the patient's overall well-being.

206. Active range of motion (AROM)

Active range of motion (AROM) in nursing refers to the degree of movement that a patient is able to achieve in a joint using their own muscle strength and without any assistance. Nurses often assess a patient's AROM to determine their level of mobility and to monitor changes in their physical condition. This assessment can help healthcare providers develop appropriate care plans and interventions to improve or maintain a patient's range of motion.

Active range of motion (AROM) assessments typically involve asking the patient to move their joints through a series of movements in different directions, such as flexion, extension, abduction, adduction, and rotation. Nurses may document the degree of movement achieved by the patient in each direction to track progress over time.

AROM assessments are important in nursing care because they provide valuable information about a patient's physical abilities, functional status, and overall musculoskeletal health. Changes in AROM can indicate improvements or declines in a patient's condition and may prompt further evaluation or interventions to prevent complications such as muscle contractures or joint stiffness.

Nurses may also use AROM assessments to educate patients on exercises and activities that can help maintain or improve their range of motion. By encouraging regular physical activity and mobility exercises, nurses can support patients in preserving their independence and enhancing their quality of life.

207. Adjuvant

An adjuvant in nursing refers to a substance or treatment that is added to a primary therapy to enhance its effectiveness. In the context of nursing care, adjuvants can include medications, therapies, or interventions that are used in conjunction with a main treatment to improve the overall outcome for the patient. Adjuvants are often employed to manage symptoms, enhance the therapeutic effect of medications, or support the body's healing process.

208. Afebrile

Afebrile in nursing means that a patient does not have a fever. Afebrile indicates that the individual's body temperature is within the normal range.

In nursing, monitoring body temperature is an essential aspect of patient care. When a patient is described as afebrile, it means that they do not currently have a fever. Normal body temperature typically ranges between 97°F to 99°F (36.1°C to 37.2°C), although it can vary depending on factors such as age, time of day, and individual variations.

When assessing a patient, nurses look for signs of fever, such as increased body temperature, chills, sweating, and general malaise. Being afebrile can indicate that the patient's body is not currently fighting an infection or experiencing an inflammatory response that would cause a fever.

If a patient was previously febrile but is now afebrile, it could indicate that their body has successfully resolved the underlying issue causing the fever. However, it is crucial for healthcare providers to continue monitoring the patient's condition to ensure that the fever does not return or that there are no other concerning developments.

209. Agglutination

Agglutination in nursing refers to the clumping together of cells or particles in the blood or other bodily fluids due to the presence of specific antibodies. This reaction is commonly used in laboratory tests to detect the presence of certain diseases or conditions, such as in blood typing or identifying infections. In nursing, agglutination tests are often performed to help diagnose and monitor various health conditions.

Agglutination tests are based on the principle of specific antibodies binding to antigens on the surface of cells or particles, causing them to clump together. This clumping reaction can be visually observed in the laboratory, indicating the presence of a specific antigen-antibody interaction. By using different reagents and techniques, healthcare providers can perform agglutination tests for a variety of purposes, including blood typing, cross-matching blood for transfusions, diagnosing infectious diseases like malaria or typhoid fever, and monitoring autoimmune conditions.

In nursing practice, understanding agglutination reactions is vital for accurate diagnosis and treatment of patients. Nurses may be involved in collecting samples, performing tests, interpreting results, and communicating findings to the healthcare team. By recognizing the significance of agglutination patterns and understanding their implications, nurses can contribute to the effective management of various medical conditions and help ensure the best possible outcomes for their patients.

210. Alopecia

Alopecia is a term used in nursing to refer to a condition that results in hair loss. It can occur in different forms and can be caused by various factors such as genetics, medical conditions, medications, or stress. Nurses may encounter patients experiencing alopecia and provide care and support to manage the condition and its effects on the individual's well-being.

Alopecia can manifest in different ways, including patchy hair loss (alopecia areata), total hair loss on the scalp (alopecia totalis), or complete hair loss across the body (alopecia universalis). It can have a significant impact on a person's self-esteem, body image, and psychological well-being. Nurses play a crucial role in educating and supporting patients with alopecia, helping them cope with the emotional aspects of hair loss, exploring treatment options, and promoting self-care practices to manage the condition. By providing compassionate care and addressing the holistic needs of individuals with alopecia, nurses contribute to enhancing their quality of life and promoting overall well-being.

211. Anaphylaxis

Anaphylaxis is a severe and potentially life-threatening allergic reaction that can occur rapidly after exposure to an allergen such as certain foods, insect venom, medications, or latex. In nursing, understanding anaphylaxis is crucial as nurses play a key role in recognizing the signs and symptoms of anaphylaxis, initiating emergency treatment including administering epinephrine, and providing ongoing care and monitoring for patients experiencing anaphylaxis. Educating patients about triggers, symptoms, and management of anaphylaxis is also an important aspect of nursing care.

Anaphylaxis is a medical emergency that requires prompt recognition and intervention. In nursing practice, nurses must be knowledgeable about the signs and symptoms of anaphylaxis, which can include difficulty breathing, swelling of the throat, hives, rapid onset of itching, flushing, and a drop in blood pressure. Nurses are trained to quickly assess patients experiencing anaphylaxis, administer epinephrine as needed, and provide supportive care such as ensuring airway patency, administering supplemental oxygen, and monitoring the patient's vital signs.

In addition to immediate management, nursing care for patients with a history of anaphylaxis includes educating them on identifying triggers, carrying an epinephrine autoinjector, and seeking prompt medical attention in case of a reaction. Nurses also collaborate with other healthcare professionals to develop individualized care plans for patients at risk of anaphylaxis, ensuring that they receive appropriate follow-up care and support.

Overall, anaphylaxis management in nursing involves a comprehensive approach that focuses on prevention, early recognition, effective treatment, and ongoing patient education to minimize the risk of future allergic reactions. Nurses play a critical role in caring for patients with anaphylaxis and promoting positive outcomes through their expertise, advocacy, and patient-centered approach.

212. Angina

Angina in nursing refers to a condition characterized by chest pain or discomfort that occurs when the heart muscle does not receive enough oxygen-rich blood. It is usually a symptom of underlying heart disease, such as coronary artery disease. Nurses play a crucial role in assessing and managing patients with angina, monitoring their symptoms, administering medications, and providing education on lifestyle changes to help manage the condition.

213. Anti-inflammatory

Anti-inflammatory in nursing refers to medications or treatments that help reduce inflammation in the body. Inflammation is a response by the immune system to injury or infection, but sometimes it can be excessive or chronic. Anti-inflammatory agents are used to relieve symptoms such as pain, swelling, and redness that result from inflammatory processes. Nurses may administer or monitor the effects of anti-inflammatory medications as part of patient care.

In nursing practice, understanding anti-inflammatory medications is crucial as they play a significant role in managing various conditions. There are two main types of anti-inflammatory drugs: non-steroidal anti-inflammatory drugs (NSAIDs) and corticosteroids. NSAIDs work by blocking the production of certain chemicals in the body that cause inflammation, thereby reducing pain and swelling. Common examples of NSAIDs include ibuprofen, naproxen, and aspirin.

Corticosteroids, on the other hand, are synthetic drugs that mimic the effects of hormones produced by the adrenal glands. They are often prescribed for more severe inflammatory conditions such as arthritis, asthma, and inflammatory bowel diseases. Corticosteroids help reduce inflammation by suppressing the immune response that triggers it.

Nurses need to assess patients for conditions that may benefit from anti-inflammatory treatment, administer medications as prescribed by healthcare providers, and monitor patients for side effects or adverse reactions. They also play a role in educating patients about the importance of taking medications as directed and following up with healthcare providers if they have any concerns.

214. Apnea

Apnea in nursing refers to the temporary cessation of breathing. This is a critical condition that requires immediate attention and intervention to ensure that the patient's breathing is restored. Apnea can be caused by various factors, such as respiratory diseases, drug overdose, or neurological problems. Nursing care for a patient with apnea may involve monitoring their vital signs, administering oxygen therapy, and assisting with interventions to help them resume breathing.

Apnea can be categorized into different types based on the duration and cause of the breathing pauses. Some common types of apnea include:

1. Central Apnea: This occurs when the brain fails to send signals to the muscles that control breathing. It is often seen in conditions like brain injuries, strokes, or certain neurological disorders.

2. Obstructive Apnea: This type of apnea happens when there is a physical blockage in the airway, preventing airflow into the lungs. It can be caused by factors such as obesity, enlarged tonsils, or a narrowed airway.

3. Mixed Apnea: This type involves a combination of central and obstructive apnea, where both brain signaling issues and airway obstructions contribute to breathing pauses.

Nurses play a crucial role in recognizing the signs of apnea, monitoring patients for breathing irregularities, and providing timely interventions. Respiratory assessments, continuous monitoring of oxygen saturation levels, and implementing appropriate interventions, such as positioning adjustments, administering medications, or initiating respiratory support like oxygen therapy or mechanical ventilation, are all essential aspects of nursing care for patients with apnea.

In addition to immediate interventions, nurses also educate patients and their families about apnea management, breathing techniques, lifestyle modifications, and the importance of follow-up care. Collaborating with other healthcare professionals, such as respiratory therapists, physicians, and sleep specialists, is key to developing comprehensive care plans tailored to each patient's unique needs and condition.

215. Arrhythmia

Arrhythmia is a medical condition characterized by an abnormal rhythm of the heart. In nursing, understanding arrhythmias is important as nurses often monitor patients for signs and symptoms of irregular heart rhythms. Nurses play a critical role in assessing, monitoring, and managing patients with arrhythmias to ensure their safety and well-being.

Arrhythmias can manifest as a variety of electrical disturbances in the heart, leading to irregular heartbeats such as tachycardia (rapid heartbeat), bradycardia (slow heartbeat), and atrial fibrillation (quivering or irregular heartbeat). Nurses need to be skilled in recognizing the signs and symptoms of arrhythmias, interpreting ECG readings, and understanding the potential causes and implications of different types of arrhythmias.

In the nursing field, managing patients with arrhythmias involves closely monitoring their heart rate and rhythm, administering medications as prescribed by the healthcare provider, and providing education to patients and their families about the condition and its management. Nurses also play a key role in collaborating with other healthcare team members, such as cardiologists and electrophysiologists, to develop and implement an appropriate care plan for patients with arrhythmias.

Furthermore, nurses need to be prepared to respond promptly in emergency situations where arrhythmias can lead to life-threatening complications such as cardiac arrest. This may involve performing interventions like administering medications, providing defibrillation, and coordinating with the healthcare team to stabilize the patient.

Overall, a thorough understanding of arrhythmias and their management is essential for nurses to deliver high-quality care to patients with cardiac rhythm abnormalities.

216. Arterial

Arterial in nursing usually refers to anything related to arteries, which are blood vessels that carry oxygenated blood away from the heart to the tissues of the body. In nursing, assessing arterial blood flow, monitoring arterial blood gases, and performing arterial blood gas sampling are some common tasks that involve dealing with arteries.

217. Atelectasis

Atelectasis in nursing refers to a condition where there is a partial or complete collapse of a lung or a section of the lung. This can occur when the tiny air sacs called alveoli within the lung deflate, leading to reduced or absent gas exchange. Atelectasis can result from various factors such as blockages in the airways, pressure on the lungs from outside the chest, or shallow breathing. Nurses play a crucial role in identifying, managing, and preventing atelectasis in patients to ensure optimal respiratory function.

218. Axilla

"Oral Axilla" is a term used in nursing to describe the practice of taking a patient's temperature by placing a thermometer in their armpit. This method is often used in situations where it may be difficult to take an oral temperature reading, such as with young children or patients who are unable to cooperate. The armpit temperature reading is slightly lower than oral temperature and is considered less accurate but convenient and non-invasive in certain situations.

Some key points to keep in mind when taking an axillary temperature include ensuring that the patient's armpit is dry before placing the thermometer, as any moisture can affect the accuracy of the reading. Additionally, the thermometer should be held in place firmly under the arm for the recommended amount of time, typically a few minutes, to ensure an accurate measurement.

While axillary temperature readings may be more convenient in certain situations, they are generally considered less accurate than oral temperature readings due to factors such as external temperature, clothing, and individual variability. In cases where precise temperature monitoring is crucial, such as in critically ill patients or when monitoring for fever, healthcare providers may opt for more accurate measurement methods like oral, rectal, or tympanic temperature readings. Consulting with a healthcare professional can help determine the most appropriate method for taking a patient's temperature based on their specific circumstances.

219. Benign

Benign in nursing refers to a condition that is not malignant or cancerous. Benign tumors or conditions are generally considered non-threatening and usually do not spread to other parts of the body. In the context of nursing, understanding the difference between benign and malignant conditions is important for providing appropriate care and treatment to patients.

Benign conditions in nursing can encompass a variety of health issues beyond just tumors. For example, benign inflammatory conditions like appendicitis can be effectively treated with surgery, resolving the issue without major long-term consequences. In nursing practice, it is crucial to accurately diagnose whether a condition is benign or malignant, as this distinction greatly influences the treatment plan and patient outcomes. By closely monitoring patients with benign conditions and providing appropriate care, nurses play a vital role in promoting healing and recovery.

220. Biohazard

In nursing, the term "biohazard" refers to any biological material that poses a threat to the health of living organisms, especially humans. This can include blood, bodily fluids, tissues, and other materials that may contain infectious microorganisms such as bacteria, viruses, or other pathogens. Nurses must handle biohazardous materials carefully to prevent the spread of infections and protect both themselves and their patients from potential harm. Proper disposal and handling procedures are essential to minimize the risk of exposure to biohazards in a healthcare setting.

Strict protocols and guidelines are in place to ensure that nurses and other healthcare workers properly manage biohazardous materials. This includes using personal protective equipment (PPE) such as gloves, gowns, masks, and eye protection when handling potentially infectious materials. Nurses are trained on how to safely collect, transport, and dispose of biohazardous waste to prevent contamination and minimize the risk of infection transmission.

In healthcare settings, biohazard symbols and labels are used to clearly identify materials that pose a biological risk. These symbols serve as a warning to alert individuals to the presence of potentially hazardous substances and remind them to take appropriate precautions.

Nurses play a critical role in preventing the spread of infections within healthcare facilities by following established protocols for handling biohazardous materials. By adhering to strict safety procedures and remaining vigilant in their handling of such materials, nurses can help protect themselves, their colleagues, and their patients from the risks associated with biological hazards.

221. Bradycardia

Bradycardia in nursing refers to a medical condition characterized by a slow heart rate, typically fewer than 60 beats per minute. In a healthcare setting, nurses monitor patients for bradycardia as it can be a sign of an underlying health issue or a side effect of certain medications. Nurses may need to intervene by notifying the healthcare team or providing appropriate treatment if bradycardia is identified in a patient.

Bradycardia can be caused by various factors, including certain medical conditions like hypothyroidism, electrolyte imbalances, heart disease, or side effects of medications such as beta-blockers. In nursing, it is crucial for healthcare professionals to recognize the signs and symptoms of bradycardia, such as dizziness, fatigue, confusion, and fainting, as it can lead to serious complications like decreased blood flow to vital organs.

Nurses play a key role in monitoring and assessing patients with bradycardia, using tools like electrocardiograms (ECGs) to accurately diagnose the condition. Depending on the severity and underlying cause of bradycardia, nurses may need to collaborate with other healthcare providers to determine the appropriate treatment plan. Interventions for bradycardia may include administering medications, adjusting current medications, or implementing more invasive treatments like pacemaker placement.

Education and patient counseling are also essential components of nursing care for patients with bradycardia. Nurses often provide valuable information to patients and their families about the condition, lifestyle modifications, medication management, and when to seek medical assistance. By closely monitoring patients with bradycardia and providing comprehensive care, nurses can help optimize patient outcomes and improve their quality of life.

222. Bronchitis

Bronchitis is an inflammation of the bronchial tubes, which are the airways that carry air to the lungs. In nursing, bronchitis refers to the condition where the bronchial tubes become inflamed, often resulting in symptoms such as coughing, chest discomfort, and difficulty breathing. Nurses may be involved in assessing patients with bronchitis, providing care, administering medications, and educating patients on managing the condition.

223. Budding

Budding in nursing usually refers to a process where a nurse who is newly qualified or in training is paired with a more experienced nurse for mentorship and guidance. This practice helps newer nurses develop their skills, knowledge, and confidence under the guidance of a more seasoned professional. It can also help in facilitating a smooth transition into the nursing profession and ensure quality patient care.

Budding in nursing is a form of mentorship that is crucial for the professional development of new nurses. It allows them to learn from experienced nurses who can provide guidance, support, and wisdom accumulated through years of practice. Through this relationship, budding nurses can enhance their clinical skills, critical thinking abilities, and decision-making processes. Additionally, the mentorship process can help budding nurses navigate the complexities of the healthcare system, understand hospital procedures, and develop a deeper understanding of patient care. Overall, budding in nursing plays a significant role in fostering a supportive and nurturing environment for new nurses as they embark on their careers in healthcare.

224. Carcinoma

Carcinoma is a type of cancer that begins in the skin or tissues that line or cover internal organs. It is a broad term that encompasses various types of cancer that originate from epithelial cells. In nursing, understanding different types of carcinoma, their symptoms, treatments, and care management is essential for providing care to patients diagnosed with this condition.

Carcinoma is the most common type of cancer diagnosed in humans. It can occur in many different organs and tissues throughout the body, including the skin, lungs, breasts, prostate, colon, and more. Carcinomas are named based on the type of cells from which they originate. For example, adenocarcinoma arises from glandular tissue, squamous cell carcinoma develops from squamous cells, and basal cell carcinoma originates from the basal cells of the skin.

Nurses play a crucial role in caring for patients with carcinoma. This includes assessing patients for signs and symptoms of cancer, providing education on treatment options and side effects, supporting patients and their families emotionally, and assisting in symptom management and palliative care. Nurses also collaborate with other members of the healthcare team to coordinate comprehensive care for patients with carcinoma, ensuring that they receive appropriate treatments and support throughout their illness.

225. Cardiopulmonary

Cardiopulmonary in nursing refers to the assessment and management of conditions affecting both the heart (cardio) and lungs (pulmonary). Nurses who specialize in cardiopulmonary care are trained to monitor and treat patients with various heart and lung disorders, such as heart failure, asthma, chronic obstructive pulmonary disease (COPD), and pneumonia. They play a crucial role in providing care, education, and support to patients with cardiopulmonary conditions to improve their overall health and well-being.

226. Chemotherapy

Chemotherapy in nursing refers to the administration of chemical drugs or medications to treat cancer. Nurses play a crucial role in chemotherapy treatment by preparing and administering the medications, monitoring patients for side effects, educating patients on the treatment regimen and managing any complications that may arise during the course of treatment. Nurses also provide emotional support to patients undergoing chemotherapy and ensure that they receive proper care and assistance throughout their treatment journey.

Chemotherapy in nursing is a complex and important aspect of cancer care. Nurses who specialize in oncology play a critical role in the delivery of chemotherapy treatment to patients. They work closely with oncologists and other healthcare providers to ensure that patients receive the correct dosage of medication, understand the potential side effects, and have their symptoms managed effectively.

In addition to administering chemotherapy drugs, nurses also monitor patients closely during treatment to assess their response to the medications and to identify any adverse reactions. They provide education to patients and their families about what to expect during treatment, how to manage side effects at home, and the importance of adhering to the prescribed treatment plan.

Nurses in chemotherapy units often develop strong relationships with their patients, providing not just medical care but also emotional support and encouragement throughout the challenging process of cancer treatment. They play a vital role in advocating for patients' needs and coordinating care to ensure the best possible outcomes.

Overall, nurses in chemotherapy care settings are instrumental in ensuring that patients receive safe, effective, and compassionate care during their cancer treatment journey.

227. Clotting

Clotting in nursing refers to the process of blood coagulation that occurs naturally in response to injury or bleeding. When a blood vessel is injured, a series of complex reactions involving platelets and clotting factors are triggered to form a blood clot and stop the bleeding. Nurses monitor clotting in patients to ensure that blood is clotting appropriately and to prevent excessive bleeding or clotting disorders. They may also administer medications such as anticoagulants or clotting factors to manage clotting disorders.

228. Colitis

Colitis in nursing refers to the inflammation of the colon (large intestine). It is a condition that can have various causes, including infections, autoimmune reactions, and inflammatory bowel diseases. Colitis can lead to symptoms such as abdominal pain, diarrhea, and bloody stools. Nurses play a crucial role in assessing and managing patients with colitis, providing care, monitoring symptoms, and collaborating with other healthcare providers for effective treatment and support to provide optimal care for patients with colitis, nurses must have a good understanding of the condition and its potential causes, symptoms, and complications. They play a key role in assessing patients, monitoring vital signs, administering medications as prescribed, and educating patients about their condition and self-care measures. Nurses also collaborate with other members of the healthcare team, including physicians, dietitians, and other specialists, to develop individualized care plans that address the unique needs of each patient.

In addition, nurses may assist in diagnostic procedures such as colonoscopies or imaging studies to help diagnose colitis and monitor its progression. They also provide emotional support to patients and their families, as living with a chronic condition like colitis can be challenging and impact a person's quality of life.

Overall, nurses in the field of gastroenterology or in settings where they care for patients with colitis must have the necessary knowledge, skills, and compassion to provide holistic care that addresses not just the physical symptoms of the condition but also the emotional and psychological aspects that patients may be experiencing.

229. Consciousness

Consciousness in nursing refers to the state of mental awareness and responsiveness of a patient. It is an important aspect of patient assessment in nursing, as it provides insights into the patient's level of alertness and ability to interact with their environment. Nurses often assess consciousness by evaluating the patient's orientation to time, place, and person, as well as their ability to follow commands and respond appropriately. Changes in consciousness may indicate underlying health issues or be a result of various factors such as medication, trauma, or illness, and it is crucial for nurses to monitor and address any alterations in a patient's consciousness to ensure their well-being.

230. Contracture

Contracture in nursing refers to the permanent shortening or tightening of muscles, tendons, or other tissues, often leading to deformity or restriction of movement. This condition can result from prolonged immobility, such as being bedridden or having limited mobility, and can be a significant concern for patients in nursing care. Nurses need to monitor patients at risk for contractures and implement interventions to prevent or manage this condition, such as range of motion exercises, positioning strategies, and the use of splints or braces.

Contractures are particularly common in patients with conditions that limit their ability to move and change positions independently, such as individuals recovering from a stroke, those with spinal cord injuries, or patients with certain neurological disorders. The lack of movement and prolonged positioning can cause the muscles to become shortened and stiff over time. As a result, contractures can lead to pain, discomfort, skin breakdown, and a reduced quality of life for patients.

Nurses play a crucial role in assessing patients for signs of developing contractures, implementing preventive measures, and managing existing contractures. Prevention strategies may include regular repositioning of bedridden patients, performing range of motion exercises, using appropriate supportive devices, and encouraging physical activity as tolerated. When contractures develop, nurses may work with other healthcare professionals, such as physical therapists, to design and implement a treatment plan that aims to improve flexibility, reduce pain, and help patients regain functional mobility.

Overall, understanding contractures and their implications is essential for nurses working in various healthcare settings, as they play a vital role in promoting patient comfort, mobility, and overall well-being.

231. CPM (continuous passive motion)

Continuous Passive Motion (CPM) is a therapy technique used in nursing and physical therapy to help with joint rehabilitation. It involves the use of a mechanical device that slowly and continuously moves a joint through a prescribed range of motion. This technique is often used after surgeries or injuries to help improve joint mobility, increase circulation, prevent stiffness, and reduce pain.

Passive Motion (CPM) machines are often used after joint surgeries, especially knee or hip surgeries, to prevent scar tissue formation and promote healing. These machines allow the joint to move in a controlled manner within a specific range of motion, without the patient actively moving the joint themselves.

The CPM machine can be adjusted to fit the patient's comfort level and rehabilitation needs. The continuous motion helps to lubricate the joint, increase the flow of synovial fluid, and prevent joint stiffness. It also aids in reducing pain and swelling associated with the surgery or injury.

Nurses and physical therapists play a crucial role in monitoring the patient's progress with CPM therapy, ensuring that the machine is set up correctly, and adjusting the settings as needed. They also educate the patient on how to use the machine safely and effectively.

Overall, Continuous Passive Motion therapy can be an important part of a patient's recovery plan after joint surgery or injury, helping to improve outcomes and speed up the rehabilitation process.

232. Cystic fibrosis

Cystic fibrosis is a genetic disorder that affects the respiratory and digestive systems. In nursing, it refers to the care and management of patients with cystic fibrosis. Nurses who work with patients with cystic fibrosis are responsible for providing support, education, and medical care to help manage the symptoms of the disease and improve the quality of life for patients. This may include administering medications, assisting with airway clearance techniques, monitoring respiratory function, and providing emotional support to patients and their families.

In nursing, caring for patients with cystic fibrosis involves a holistic approach that addresses both the physical and emotional needs of the patient. Nurses play a crucial role in educating patients and their families about the disease, treatment options, and self-care techniques. They also work closely with other healthcare professionals to develop and implement individualized care plans that address the unique needs of each patient.

Nurses often help patients with cystic fibrosis manage their symptoms through various interventions such as chest physiotherapy, exercise programs, nutritional support, and medication administration. They also monitor patients' respiratory status, perform assessments to evaluate their condition, and communicate any changes to the healthcare team.

Caring for patients with cystic fibrosis can be challenging due to the chronic nature of the disease and the impact it has on patients' daily lives. Nurses in this field must be compassionate, knowledgeable, and dedicated to providing high-quality care to help patients manage their symptoms and improve their quality of life.

233. Decubitus

Decubitus in nursing refers to a pressure ulcer, which is also known as a bedsore. It is a type of wound that develops when an area of the skin and underlying tissue is subject to prolonged pressure or friction. Decubitus ulcers commonly occur in bedridden or immobile patients, particularly in areas where bones are close to the skin surface, such as the heels, hips, and tailbone. It is crucial for nurses to prevent and manage decubitus ulcers to promote patient comfort and prevent complications.

To reposition the patient regularly to relieve pressure on vulnerable areas, ensuring proper nutrition and hydration to promote tissue healing, using appropriate support surfaces such as special mattresses or cushions, and maintaining skin cleanliness and dryness. Nurses play a critical role in assessing, preventing, and managing decubitus ulcers to provide the best possible care for their patients. By following evidence-based practices and guidelines, nurses can help prevent the development of pressure ulcers and promote the healing of existing wounds. It is essential for healthcare providers to collaborate with the nursing team to develop comprehensive care plans tailored to each patient's needs in order to prevent decubitus ulcers and improve patient outcomes.

234. Delirium

Delirium in the nursing context refers to a sudden state of confusion or changes in mental status that can occur in patients, particularly in older adults or those with underlying health conditions. It is often characterized by disturbances in attention, awareness, and cognition. Delirium can have various causes such as infections, medication side effects, dehydration, or other medical conditions. Nurses play a crucial role in assessing, managing, and monitoring patients with delirium to ensure their safety and well-being.

Delirium is a serious condition that can have significant implications for patient outcomes if not promptly recognized and managed. It is crucial for nurses to be skilled in assessing patients for symptoms of delirium, which can include confusion, agitation, disorientation, hallucinations, and altered levels of consciousness. Nurses may use specific assessment tools to evaluate the severity of delirium and track changes over time.

In nursing practice, addressing delirium involves identifying and treating the underlying causes, such as infections, metabolic imbalances, medication effects, or environmental factors. Nurses may work with other healthcare professionals to develop a comprehensive care plan tailored to the individual patient's needs. This plan may include interventions to help prevent complications, promote safety, and support the patient's comfort and well-being.

Furthermore, nurses play a vital role in educating patients, family members, and caregivers about delirium, its potential causes, and the importance of early intervention. By raising awareness and providing information, nurses can help empower others to recognize the signs of delirium and seek appropriate medical attention promptly.

Overall, delirium is a complex and multifaceted condition that requires a coordinated and interdisciplinary approach to care. Nurses' expertise in assessment, communication, and intervention is instrumental in optimizing outcomes for patients experiencing delirium and ensuring their journey to recovery.

235. Disinfectant

Disinfectant in nursing refers to a chemical substance used to kill or inhibit the growth of microorganisms on surfaces. In a healthcare setting, disinfectants are crucial for preventing the spread of infections. Nurses use disinfectants to clean and sanitize various surfaces, medical equipment, and instruments to maintain a safe and hygienic environment for patients and healthcare providers.

Disinfectants in nursing play a critical role in infection control practices by effectively eliminating harmful bacteria, viruses, and other pathogens that can cause illnesses. Nurses use disinfectants in various healthcare settings, such as hospitals, clinics, nursing homes, and ambulatory care facilities, to reduce the risk of healthcare-associated infections.

Different types of disinfectants are used in nursing, including quaternary ammonium compounds, chlorine-based disinfectants, alcohols, hydrogen peroxide, and phenolic compounds. Each type of disinfectant has specific properties and is designed to target different pathogens. Nurses follow strict protocols and guidelines when using disinfectants to ensure proper disinfection and prevent the development of resistance in bacteria.

In the context of nursing practice, understanding the proper use of disinfectants, including the appropriate concentration, contact time, and application methods, is essential for maintaining a clean and safe healthcare environment. By effectively employing disinfectants, nurses can help reduce the risk of infections and promote patient safety and well-being.

236. Distension

Distension in nursing generally refers to the abnormal enlargement or ballooning of an organ or structure within the body. It can refer to a bloated or swollen appearance of a particular body part, often indicating an underlying issue or condition. In a medical context, nurses may assess and monitor for signs of distension as part of their patient care to detect any potential health concerns.

Distension can occur in various parts of the body, such as the abdomen (abdominal distension), the bladder (bladder distension), or other organs. Nursing assessments for distension may involve observing the affected area for changes in size, shape, or appearance, as well as evaluating the patient's symptoms and vital signs. Nursing interventions for distension may include providing comfort measures, monitoring fluid intake and output, assisting with mobility as needed, and collaborating with other healthcare providers for further evaluation and treatment. Prompt recognition and management of distension are crucial in nursing care to ensure the best outcomes for patients.

237. Diurese

Diuresis in nursing refers to the process of increasing urine production by the kidneys. This can be achieved through the administration of diuretic medications or other interventions to help remove excess fluid and waste from the body. Diuresis is often used in the management of conditions such as heart failure, kidney disease, and certain types of edema to help reduce fluid overload and improve overall health.

Diuresis is an important nursing concept because it plays a crucial role in maintaining fluid balance and managing various health conditions. By promoting diuresis, healthcare providers aim to help the body eliminate excess fluid, waste products, and electrolytes, which can accumulate due to conditions such as heart failure, kidney disease, liver disease, and certain medications. Diuretic medications are commonly used to induce diuresis by altering the function of the kidneys, leading to increased urine production.

Nurses play a key role in monitoring diuresis in patients by assessing factors such as urine output, fluid intake, electrolyte levels, and signs of dehydration or fluid overload. Close monitoring is essential to ensure that diuresis is occurring effectively without causing harmful imbalances in the body's fluid and electrolyte levels. Nurses also educate patients about the importance of complying with prescribed diuretic regimens, maintaining adequate fluid intake, and recognizing signs of potential complications related to diuresis.

In addition to medication management, nurses may use other strategies to promote diuresis in patients, such as encouraging physical activity, optimizing fluid intake, and adjusting dietary sodium intake. Through these interventions, nurses help support the body's natural mechanisms for regulating fluid balance and promoting overall health and well-being.

238. Dorsiflexion

Dorsiflexion in nursing refers to the movement of bending the foot upward at the ankle joint, bringing the top of the foot closer to the shin. This movement is opposite to plantar flexion, which is the movement of pointing the foot downward at the ankle joint. Dorsiflexion is an important movement in nursing care as it can help prevent foot drop and maintain range of motion in patients who are bedridden or have limited mobility.

239. Dysphagia

Dysphagia in nursing refers to difficulty or discomfort in swallowing, which can be caused by a variety of medical conditions. Nurses must be able to recognize the signs and symptoms of dysphagia in their patients to ensure they receive the proper care and treatment. Patients with dysphagia may have difficulty swallowing liquids, solids, or both, which can lead to complications such as malnutrition, dehydration, and aspiration pneumonia. Nursing interventions for dysphagia may include modifying food and liquid consistencies, providing feeding assistance, and collaborating with other healthcare professionals to develop an appropriate treatment plan.

240. Edentulous

Edentulous in nursing refers to a patient who is completely without teeth. The term is used to describe an individual who has lost all of their natural teeth. It is important for healthcare providers, including nurses, to be aware of a patient's edentulous status as it can impact the individual's oral health, ability to eat, and overall well-being.

Edentulous patients may face challenges related to chewing, digestion, speech, and self-esteem. In nursing care, it is essential to assess the oral health of edentulous patients regularly, support proper oral hygiene practices, and provide appropriate interventions to address any issues that may arise due to the absence of natural teeth. Nurses may also need to collaborate with other healthcare professionals, such as dentists or prosthodontists, to ensure that edentulous patients receive the necessary care and support to maintain their oral health and overall quality of life.

241. Endoscopy

Endoscopy in nursing refers to a medical procedure in which a flexible tube with a light and camera attached to it, known as an endoscope, is used to visually examine the interior of a hollow organ or cavity within the body. Endoscopy allows healthcare providers to diagnose and treat conditions within the gastrointestinal tract, respiratory system, urinary system, and other areas without the need for surgery. Nurses play an essential role in assisting with endoscopic procedures, providing patient care, monitoring vital signs, and ensuring patient comfort and safety throughout the process.

242. Erythrocyte

Erythrocyte in nursing refers to red blood cells, which are responsible for carrying oxygen from the lungs to the rest of the body's tissues and organs. Erythrocytes are an essential component of the circulatory system and play a crucial role in maintaining overall health and function. Nurses often monitor erythrocyte levels as part of routine blood tests to assess a patient's overall health status.

Erythrocytes, commonly known as red blood cells, are specialized cells that make up a significant portion of the blood. Their primary function is to carry oxygen from the lungs to the body's tissues and organs and transport carbon dioxide back to the lungs for exhalation. Erythrocytes are produced in the bone marrow and have a distinct disk-like shape that allows for efficient transportation of gases through narrow blood vessels.

In nursing practice, monitoring erythrocyte levels is essential for assessing a patient's overall health and detecting various medical conditions such as anemia, dehydration, and other blood disorders. Nurses are responsible for collecting blood samples, interpreting laboratory results related to erythrocyte count, hemoglobin levels, and hematocrit, and collaboratively developing care plans based on these findings.

Understanding the significance of erythrocytes in maintaining proper oxygenation and circulation is crucial for nurses to provide holistic care to patients. By recognizing changes in erythrocyte levels and addressing underlying issues promptly, nurses can help promote optimal health and well-being in their patients.

243. Essential oils

Essential oils in nursing typically refer to the use of concentrated plant extracts to promote health and well-being in a nursing or healthcare setting. Essential oils are often used in complementary and alternative medicine practices to help manage symptoms, reduce stress, improve mood, and promote relaxation. In nursing, essential oils may be used in aromatherapy, massage therapy, or other holistic approaches to care for patients. It's important for nurses to have a good understanding of the properties and potential benefits of essential oils, as well as any contraindications or safety considerations when using them with patients.

244. Excretion

Excretion in nursing refers to the process by which waste products and excess substances are eliminated from the body. This includes the removal of metabolic waste, toxins, and excess fluids through various organs such as the kidneys, liver, lungs, and skin. Nurses play a crucial role in monitoring and assisting patients with excretory functions to maintain overall health and well-being.

In nursing practice, understanding excretion is essential because it is a vital aspect of ensuring the body maintains proper balance and functions optimally. Nurses frequently assess patients' excretory functions by monitoring parameters such as urine output, bowel movements, and respiratory status.

Excretion involves several key organs and systems in the body:

1. **Kidneys**: The kidneys filter blood, remove waste products (such as urea and creatinine), and regulate the balance of electrolytes and fluids in the body. Nurses often monitor kidney function through laboratory tests like blood urea nitrogen (BUN) and creatinine levels.

2. **Liver**: The liver plays a role in metabolizing toxins and drugs, converting them into forms that can be excreted by the body. Nurses need to be aware of potential liver dysfunction that can impact excretory functions.

3. **Lungs**: The lungs help eliminate carbon dioxide, a waste product of cellular respiration. Nurses monitor respiratory status to ensure proper gas exchange and elimination of carbon dioxide.

4. **Skin**: The skin plays a role in excreting small amounts of waste products through sweat. In conditions like burns or certain skin diseases, the skin's excretory functions may be affected, and nurses must provide appropriate care.

5. **Intestines**: The intestines help eliminate waste through bowel movements. Nurses assess patients' bowel habits and provide interventions to promote regular and healthy bowel function.

By understanding the excretory functions of the body and how they can be affected by various health conditions, nurses can effectively assess, monitor, and intervene to support patients' overall health and well-being. Monitoring and assisting with excretion are vital aspects of nursing care that contribute to maintaining homeostasis and optimal functioning of the body.

245. Expectorate

Expectorate refers to the act of coughing up and spitting out material from the throat or lungs, such as mucus or phlegm. In a nursing context, expectorate may be used to describe the action or process of helping a patient clear their airways by coughing up and expelling secretions. This helps improve breathing and prevent complications such as pneumonia.

Expectoration is an important clinical assessment in nursing, especially for patients with respiratory conditions like pneumonia, bronchitis, or cystic fibrosis. Nurses may provide care interventions to promote expectoration, such as encouraging deep breathing exercises, administering medications to help loosen secretions, or using chest physiotherapy techniques to assist with clearing the airways. Effective expectoration can help improve oxygenation and prevent respiratory complications in patients with compromised lung function. Nurses play a crucial role in monitoring the quality and quantity of expectorated material to assess the patient's respiratory status and response to treatment.

246. Fasting

Fasting in nursing refers to the practice of abstaining from food and drink for a specified period before certain medical procedures or surgeries. This is done to ensure that the patient's stomach is empty, which can help prevent complications during the procedure, such as aspiration of stomach contents. In nursing practice, it is important to follow specific fasting guidelines provided by healthcare providers to ensure patient safety and well-being.

Fasting in nursing is a critical aspect of patient care that is often necessary before procedures like surgery, diagnostic tests, or certain treatments. Healthcare providers typically provide detailed instructions to patients regarding the specific time frames for fasting, which may include restrictions on eating, drinking, and sometimes even medications.

Fasting periods can vary depending on the procedure being performed and the patient's individual health status. For example, patients may be asked to fast for several hours before surgery to reduce the risk of complications like aspiration pneumonia. In some cases, patients may need to fast overnight before a procedure that requires general anesthesia.

Nurses play a crucial role in educating patients about the importance of fasting and ensuring that they adhere to the fasting guidelines provided by the healthcare team. They also closely monitor patients to assess their nutritional status, hydration levels, and overall well-being during the fasting period.

Overall, fasting in nursing is a key aspect of patient safety and care that helps minimize the risk of complications and ensures successful outcomes for various medical procedures and interventions.

247. Fistula

A fistula in nursing refers to an abnormal connection or passageway that forms between two organs or between an organ and the skin. In medical contexts, fistulas are often considered a complication of surgeries, injuries, or diseases. In nursing, managing fistulas typically involves wound care, monitoring for signs of infection, assisting in drainage, and providing patient education on managing the condition. Fistulas can be classified based on their location, such as rectovaginal fistulas (connecting the rectum and vagina), arteriovenous fistulas (connecting an artery and vein), or enterocutaneous fistulas (connecting the intestines to the skin). These abnormal connections can result in various symptoms like pain, infection, abscess formation, and abnormal drainage. Nursing care for patients with fistulas involves providing physical and emotional support, ensuring proper hygiene, monitoring for complications, assisting in wound management, and collaborating with the healthcare team to promote healing and overall well-being. Patient education on self-care, diet, and lifestyle modifications is also essential in managing fistulas effectively.

248. Gentian violet

Gentian violet, also known as crystal violet, is a purple dye with antifungal and antibacterial properties. In nursing, it is sometimes used topically to treat certain skin infections, oral thrush in infants, and to mark anatomic landmarks on the skin for surgical procedures. It is important for nurses to follow appropriate protocols and guidelines when using gentian violet to ensure patient safety and effectiveness of treatment.

Gentian violet is typically used in nursing settings for its antifungal properties. It works by interfering with fungal cell membranes and preventing their growth and reproduction. When used topically, it can help treat certain skin infections caused by fungi, such as ringworm or fungal diaper rash. Gentian violet may also be used to treat oral thrush in infants, a common fungal infection characterized by white patches in the mouth. Additionally, in some cases, nurses may use gentian violet to mark anatomical landmarks on the skin before surgical procedures to help guide the surgical team.

While gentian violet can be effective in treating fungal infections, it is important for nurses to be cautious when using it due to its staining properties. Gentian violet can leave a purple stain on the skin and clothing, which may be difficult to remove. Nurses should ensure proper application techniques and advise patients on how to manage any staining that occurs. Furthermore, it is essential to follow recommended dosages and guidelines to prevent adverse reactions or side effects.

Overall, gentian violet is a useful tool in nursing practice for treating fungal infections and marking skin for surgical procedures. When used correctly and with proper care, gentian violet can be a valuable treatment option in various clinical settings.

249. Geriatric

The term "geriatric" in nursing refers to the branch of healthcare focused on providing care for elderly individuals. Geriatric nursing involves meeting the unique physical, mental, and emotional needs of older adults in various healthcare settings, such as hospitals, nursing homes, and assisted living facilities. Geriatric nurses are trained to address age-related conditions, promote wellness, and enhance the quality of life for elderly patients.

250. Granulation

Granulation in nursing refers to the process of new blood vessels and connective tissue forming in a wound as part of the healing process. Granulation tissue typically appears pink or red and consists of small bumps or nodules. This is a normal part of the wound healing process and indicates that the wound is progressing towards closure. Nurses often monitor granulation tissue as part of wound care management to ensure that the wound is healing properly.

Granulation tissue plays a crucial role in the wound healing process by filling in the wound bed and providing a scaffold for the formation of new skin cells. It is rich in blood vessels, fibroblasts, and collagen, which help facilitate the growth of new tissue and promote wound closure. Granulation tissue usually forms in the proliferative phase of wound healing, following the inflammatory phase where the initial injury response takes place.

Nurses assess granulation tissue as part of their wound care management duties to ensure that the wound is healing properly. They look for characteristics such as color, size, and amount of granulation tissue present, as well as any signs of infection or abnormal healing. Proper wound care techniques, including keeping the wound clean and moist, may help promote the formation of healthy granulation tissue and facilitate the overall healing process.

Understanding the role of granulation tissue in wound healing is essential for nurses to provide effective care and support to patients with various types of wounds, such as surgical incisions, pressure ulcers, or burns. By monitoring and assessing granulation tissue, nurses can identify any issues that may impede the healing process and take appropriate actions to promote optimal wound healing.

251. Hemostasis

Hemostasis in nursing refers to the process of controlling bleeding to promote the cessation of blood flow and maintain vascular integrity. Nurses play a crucial role in assessing, managing, and monitoring patients with hemostasis issues, such as those with bleeding disorders or undergoing surgery. Nurses may administer medications, apply pressure dressings, monitor vital signs, and provide education on bleeding precautions to promote optimal patient outcomes.

Hemostasis in nursing is a vital aspect of patient care, particularly in settings where bleeding control is essential, such as in surgical units, emergency departments, and critical care units. Nurses must have a thorough understanding of the physiological processes involved in hemostasis to effectively assess and manage patients with bleeding disorders or those at risk of excessive bleeding.

Nurses play a crucial role in preventing complications related to hemostasis, such as hemorrhage or thrombosis. They collaborate with healthcare providers to develop and implement individualized care plans for patients based on their specific hemostasis needs. This may involve administering medications to promote clotting, monitoring coagulation parameters, and providing patient education on signs of bleeding complications.

In addition to clinical interventions, nurses also provide emotional support and education to patients and their families regarding hemostasis management. This may include teaching patients about the importance of compliance with prescribed treatments, recognizing signs of bleeding or clotting issues, and implementing strategies to minimize the risk of injury or bleeding episodes.

Overall, hemostasis is a critical component of nursing care that requires thorough assessment, skilled intervention, and ongoing monitoring to ensure optimal patient outcomes. Nurses play a key role in promoting hemostasis and preventing complications related to bleeding disorders, ultimately contributing to improved patient safety and quality of care.

252. Hyperglycemia

Hyperglycemia in nursing refers to a condition where there is an abnormally high level of glucose (sugar) in the blood. It is commonly seen in patients with diabetes, but can also occur in individuals without diabetes due to various reasons such as stress, illness, certain medications, or other medical conditions. In nursing practice, monitoring blood glucose levels, understanding the signs and symptoms of hyperglycemia, and addressing the condition promptly are key aspects of managing this condition to prevent complications.

Hyperglycemia can lead to various complications if not managed effectively. In nursing care, it is important to closely monitor the patient's blood glucose levels through regular testing and to assess for symptoms such as increased thirst, frequent urination, blurred vision, and fatigue. Nurses need to work closely with other healthcare professionals to develop individualized care plans that may include dietary modifications, medication adjustments, and lifestyle changes to help control blood sugar levels.

In treating hyperglycemia, nurses may administer insulin or oral medications as prescribed, closely monitor the patient's response to treatment, and provide education to both the patient and their family on self-care practices to help prevent future episodes of hyperglycemia. Additionally, nurses play a crucial role in patient education, emphasizing the importance of adherence to treatment plans, regular monitoring of blood glucose levels, and seeking medical attention promptly if symptoms worsen or complications arise.

Overall, managing hyperglycemia in nursing requires a multidisciplinary approach that focuses on comprehensive care, patient education, and close monitoring to help patients effectively control their blood sugar levels and prevent further health complications.

253. Hypoglycemia

Hypoglycemia in nursing refers to a medical condition characterized by low levels of glucose (sugar) in the blood. It is a common concern for nurses, especially when caring for patients with diabetes who are taking medications that can lower blood sugar levels too much. Symptoms of hypoglycemia can include shakiness, sweating, confusion, dizziness, and in severe cases, seizures or loss of consciousness. Nurses should be trained to recognize these symptoms and provide appropriate care, such as administering glucose and closely monitoring the patient's condition.

Hypoglycemia is a critical condition that requires prompt recognition and intervention by nurses to prevent complications. The management of hypoglycemia in nursing involves assessing the patient's symptoms, checking their blood glucose levels, and providing treatment accordingly. Nurses may administer glucose tablets, glucagon injections, or intravenous dextrose to raise the patient's blood sugar levels quickly.

In addition to acute interventions, nurses play a crucial role in educating patients with diabetes about the risk factors and signs of hypoglycemia. They may provide guidance on proper medication management, monitoring blood sugar levels, and adopting lifestyle changes to prevent episodes of low blood sugar.

Moreover, nurses must be vigilant in monitoring patients at risk for hypoglycemia, such as those on insulin therapy or certain oral medications. Regular blood glucose monitoring, especially during mealtimes and periods of increased physical activity, can help prevent hypoglycemic episodes and promote better diabetes management.

Overall, nurses play a vital role in the prevention, identification, and management of hypoglycemia in patients with diabetes, ensuring their safety and well-being.

254. Ileostomy

Ileostomy in nursing refers to a surgical procedure where the ileum (the last part of the small intestine) is brought through an opening in the abdomen to create a stoma. This allows waste to bypass the colon and exit the body through the stoma into a pouch or bag worn on the outside of the body. Ileostomies are often performed as a treatment for certain medical conditions, such as inflammatory bowel disease, colon cancer, or trauma to the intestines. Nurses play a crucial role in caring for patients with an ileostomy by providing education, support, and monitoring for any complications.

255. Induration

Induration in nursing refers to the hardening of a specific area of tissue, typically due to inflammation, infection, or the formation of scar tissue. In nursing, induration can be assessed by palpation (feeling the area by touch) to determine the extent and nature of the hardening. This assessment finding can provide important information to healthcare providers about the underlying condition and can help guide further treatment.

256. Ingestion

In nursing, ingestion refers to the process of taking in food or fluids through the mouth. It is an important aspect of assessing a patient's nutritional status and overall health. Nurses often monitor and evaluate a patient's ability to ingest food and fluids properly as part of their care.

In the nursing context, ingestion is a fundamental component of assessing a patient's nutritional intake and overall well-being. Nurses play a critical role in observing and evaluating a patient's ability to ingest food and fluids effectively. This process involves not only the physical act of eating and drinking, but also monitoring the patient's intake, considering any dietary restrictions or modifications, and addressing issues such as swallowing difficulties or dysphagia.

Nurses may also assess the patient's appetite, chewing and swallowing abilities, any pain or discomfort related to eating, as well as any changes in weight or nutritional status. Proper nutrition is essential for healing, recovery, and overall health, so monitoring and supporting a patient's ingestion habits is a key aspect of nursing care.

In some cases, nurses may need to provide education to patients and their families on proper nutrition, meal planning, and strategies to improve ingestion habits. They may also collaborate with other healthcare professionals, such as dietitians or speech therapists, to develop comprehensive care plans for patients with specific nutritional needs or swallowing issues.

Overall, ingestion in nursing encompasses a range of assessments, interventions, and support mechanisms to ensure that patients are receiving adequate nutrition and hydration to support their health and well-being.

257. Inguinal

"Inguinal" in nursing refers to a body part or area of the body related to the groin. It specifically pertains to the inguinal region, which is the area where the abdomen meets the thigh. Inguinal hernias, for example, are common surgical conditions that occur when tissue, such as the intestine, protrudes through a weakened area in the abdominal wall in the inguinal region.

The inguinal region is important in nursing assessments and care since it can be a site for various health issues. In addition to inguinal hernias, nurses may also evaluate the inguinal area for lymph nodes, which can be enlarged in cases of infection or malignancy. For example, swollen inguinal lymph nodes can be a sign of a sexually transmitted infection or cancer.

Nurses must be knowledgeable about the anatomy and common conditions related to the inguinal region to provide comprehensive care to their patients. Assessing and documenting findings accurately in this area can help healthcare providers diagnose and treat conditions effectively. Proper nursing care in cases involving the inguinal region, such as wound care after surgery for an inguinal hernia repair, is crucial for promoting optimal patient outcomes.

258. Inotropic

Inotropic in nursing refers to the effect of a medication or treatment on the strength of the heart's contractions. Inotropic agents are drugs that can either increase or decrease the force of the heart's contractions. Positive inotropes increase the strength of the heart's contractions, while negative inotropes decrease the strength of the contractions. These medications are used in various clinical settings to treat conditions such as heart failure, cardiac arrhythmias, and shock.

Inotropic agents work by influencing the levels of calcium inside the heart muscle cells, which in turn affects the heart's ability to contract. Positive inotropic agents help the heart pump more effectively, which can be beneficial in conditions where the heart is not pumping with enough force, such as in heart failure. These agents can improve cardiac output and increase blood flow to the body's tissues.

On the other hand, negative inotropic agents reduce the force of the heart's contractions. They are often used in conditions like hypertension, where decreasing the heart's workload can be beneficial. By reducing the heart's contractility, negative inotropic agents can help lower blood pressure and reduce the heart's oxygen demand.

It's important for nurses to understand the effects of inotropic medications, as they play a crucial role in managing patients with cardiovascular conditions. Monitoring the patient's response to inotropic therapy, assessing for side effects, and maintaining hemodynamic stability are key components of nursing care when administering these medications.

259. Iontophoresis

Iontophoresis in nursing is a method used to deliver medication into the body through the skin using a small electric current. This technique is often used in physical therapy and wound care to administer medications such as corticosteroids, lidocaine, or other drugs to specific areas of the body. Iontophoresis can be helpful in managing conditions such as inflammation, pain, or skin disorders.

Iontophoresis works by utilizing the principle of electromigration, where an electric current is applied to facilitate the movement of charged ions, such as medication molecules, through the skin. By placing medication-containing patches or solutions on the skin near the target area and applying a low-level electrical current, iontophoresis can enhance the delivery of the medication into the underlying tissues.

In nursing practice, iontophoresis can be beneficial for reducing pain and inflammation in conditions like tendinitis, bursitis, and certain musculoskeletal injuries. It is considered a non-invasive and relatively painless method of drug administration compared to injections or oral medications. Nurses who perform iontophoresis must be trained in the technique to ensure proper application and dosage of medications as prescribed by healthcare providers.

Overall, iontophoresis can be a valuable tool for nurses in managing various patient conditions and promoting effective drug delivery while minimizing systemic side effects often associated with oral medications.

260. Irrigate

Irrigating in nursing typically refers to the process of cleansing a wound or body cavity with a fluid solution. This method is used to remove debris, control infection, and promote healing. The irrigation process involves using a syringe or other method to gently flush the area with a sterile solution such as saline.

Irrigation in nursing is a common and essential procedure used to clean wounds, surgical sites, or body cavities such as the bladder or colon. The process involves flushing the area with a sterile solution to remove debris, bacteria, and other contaminants that could hinder the healing process or lead to infection. In wound care, irrigation helps to promote healing by creating a clean environment for the body to repair itself. Nurses must be trained in proper irrigation techniques to ensure the procedure is carried out safely and effectively.

261. Keloid

A keloid is a type of raised scar that occurs when the body overreacts to an injury or wound. It can be firm, shiny, and often larger than the original wound. In nursing, keloids may be a concern when assessing and managing scars in patients.

Keloids can form anywhere on the body but are most common on the chest, shoulders, earlobes, and cheeks. They can be itchy, tender, or even painful. Keloids are more common in people with darker skin tones and are often a result of an abnormal healing response to skin injuries, such as surgical incisions, acne scars, burns, vaccinations, or body piercings.

In nursing practice, it is important for nurses to educate patients about keloids, including risk factors, preventive measures, and available treatment options. Treatment approaches may include corticosteroid injections, silicone sheets, cryotherapy, laser therapy, or surgical removal. Nurses play a role in providing wound care, monitoring for complications, and supporting patients in the management of keloids to improve their quality of life.

262. Ketones

Ketones in nursing typically refer to the presence of ketone bodies in the urine or blood of a patient. Ketones are produced when the body breaks down fats for energy in the absence of sufficient glucose. In nursing practice, detecting ketones can be important, especially in patients with conditions like diabetes, as it can indicate a state of metabolic imbalance or insufficient insulin. Monitoring ketone levels is important as high levels of ketones can lead to a serious condition called ketoacidosis.

263. Liposuction

Liposuction is a surgical procedure in which fat is removed from different parts of the body using a suction technique. It is typically done for cosmetic reasons to sculpt or contour specific areas of the body where fat accumulates, such as the abdomen, thighs, buttocks, hips, arms, or face. In nursing, liposuction may involve assisting the surgeon during the procedure, providing post-operative care to patients, monitoring their recovery, and educating them about how to care for themselves after the surgery.

264. Lumpectomy

A lumpectomy is a surgical procedure in which a surgeon removes a tumor or lump (along with a margin of surrounding tissue) from a patient's breast while preserving as much healthy breast tissue as possible. This procedure is commonly used to treat breast cancer or other breast abnormalities. Lumpectomy is also known as breast-conserving surgery because it aims to remove the tumor while maintaining the cosmetic appearance of the breast as much as possible.

265. Lymphatic

The lymphatic system in nursing refers to a network of vessels, nodes, and organs that work together to help defend the body against infections and diseases. This system plays a crucial role in maintaining fluid balance, transporting lymph (a clear fluid containing white blood cells) throughout the body, and filtering out harmful substances. Nurses often assess the lymphatic system as part of a patient's physical examination to identify signs of infection, inflammation, or other health issues.

266. Macular degeneration

Macular degeneration, also known as age-related macular degeneration (AMD), is a common eye condition that affects the central part of the retina, called the macula. This condition can cause a loss of vision in the center of the visual field, leading to difficulty with tasks like reading, driving, and recognizing faces. In nursing, understanding macular degeneration is important for providing appropriate care and support to patients who are affected by this condition. Nurses may assist patients with managing their symptoms, accessing treatment options, and making lifestyle adjustments to cope with the changes in vision caused by macular degeneration.

267. Mammogram

A mammogram is a type of breast imaging procedure used in medicine to detect and diagnose breast conditions, including breast cancer. In nursing, nurses may provide guidance and support to patients undergoing mammograms, explain the procedure to them, discuss the importance of breast health screening, and assist in the care of patients during and after the mammogram. Nurses play a crucial role in helping patients understand the purpose of mammograms and ensuring they feel comfortable and informed throughout the process.

268. Mastectomy

Mastectomy is a surgical procedure in which one or both breasts are removed, usually as a treatment for breast cancer or as a preventive measure for individuals at high risk of developing breast cancer. There are different types of mastectomies, including total mastectomy (removal of the entire breast), partial mastectomy (removal of part of the breast), and radical mastectomy (removal of the breast tissue, chest muscles, and lymph nodes). After a mastectomy, patients may undergo breast reconstruction surgery to restore the shape of the breast. Nursing care for a patient who has undergone a mastectomy includes providing support, education, wound care, pain management, and emotional support.

269. Melanoma

Melanoma in nursing refers to a type of skin cancer that originates from melanocytes, the pigment-producing cells in the skin. Nurses play a crucial role in assessing skin lesions, educating patients about skin cancer prevention, assisting in the diagnosis and treatment of melanoma, and providing support to patients and their families throughout the process. Early detection and intervention are essential in improving the prognosis and outcomes for individuals with melanoma.

Melanoma is a serious and potentially life-threatening form of skin cancer that can spread rapidly if not detected and treated early. In nursing, understanding the signs and symptoms of melanoma is crucial for conducting thorough skin assessments and identifying suspicious lesions. Nurses also play a vital role in educating patients about the importance of sun protection, regular skin checks, and seeking medical attention for any concerning changes in moles or skin pigmentation.

In addition to patient education and assessment, nurses may assist in the diagnosis of melanoma by collaborating with healthcare providers to perform biopsies or refer patients to dermatologists for further evaluation. They also provide emotional support and counseling to patients and their families, helping them navigate the emotional and psychological challenges that come with a cancer diagnosis.

Furthermore, nurses are involved in the comprehensive care of patients with melanoma, including monitoring for side effects of treatment, coordinating follow-up appointments, and promoting adherence to treatment plans. By working collaboratively with the healthcare team, nurses contribute to the holistic care of individuals with melanoma, aiming to improve outcomes and quality of life for these patients.

270. MRSA (methicillin-resistant Staphylococcus aureus)

MRSA (methicillin-resistant Staphylococcus aureus) in nursing refers to a type of staph infection caused by a strain of Staphylococcus aureus bacteria that has developed resistance to certain antibiotics, including methicillin. In nursing, MRSA is a significant concern because it can be easily transmitted from patient to patient and from healthcare workers to patients. Nurses play a crucial role in preventing the spread of MRSA by practicing good hygiene, following proper infection control protocols, and monitoring patients for signs of infection. It is important for nurses to be aware of MRSA and take appropriate precautions to prevent its spread in healthcare settings.

271. Mesenteric tube

A nasoenteric tube in nursing refers to a tube that is inserted through the nose and advanced into the small intestine to provide enteral nutrition, administer medications, drain fluids, or decompress the stomach. This type of tube is commonly used in healthcare settings to support patients who are unable to eat or digest food normally. Nasoenteric tubes are typically thinner than nasogastric tubes and are designed to reach the small intestine for more targeted delivery of nutrients or medications.

A nasoenteric tube is inserted through the nose, passed through the esophagus, and positioned in the small intestine, such as the jejunum or the duodenum. This placement allows for the direct delivery of nutrients into the small intestine, bypassing the stomach. Nasoenteric tubes are used when patients have issues with gastric motility, gastric reflux, or other gastrointestinal conditions that make it difficult for them to tolerate feeding into the stomach.

In nursing, the care of patients with nasoenteric tubes includes monitoring tube placement, assessing for any signs of complications (such as aspiration, tube dislodgement, or tube blockage), providing proper tube care, and ensuring that the prescribed feedings or medications are administered correctly. Nurses also play a crucial role in educating patients and their families on how to manage the nasoenteric tube at home, including techniques for feeding, flushing the tube, and preventing infections.

Overall, nasoenteric tubes are important tools in healthcare for supporting patients who have difficulty with oral intake or digestion, and it is essential for nursing professionals to have a thorough understanding of their use, maintenance, and potential complications in order to provide safe and effective care to patients with these tubes.

272. Neuralgia

Neuralgia in nursing refers to a condition characterized by severe, sharp, shooting, or burning pain along a nerve. It occurs when a nerve is damaged or irritated due to various factors such as infection, inflammation, compression, or injury. Nurses may encounter patients with neuralgia and are responsible for assessing their symptoms, providing appropriate care, and assisting in managing their pain through medications, therapies, or referrals to specialists as needed.

to support patients with neuralgia, nurses may also educate them on self-care techniques to manage their symptoms better. This may include advice on lifestyle changes, stress reduction strategies, and techniques for pain management, such as relaxation exercises or hot/cold therapy. Nurses play a crucial role in advocating for patients with neuralgia, ensuring they receive the necessary support and resources to improve their quality of life. By providing compassionate care and promoting holistic well-being, nurses can help patients with neuralgia cope with their condition more effectively.

273. NSAID (non-steroidal anti-inflammatory drug)

NSAID stands for non-steroidal anti-inflammatory drug. In nursing, NSAIDs are medications that help reduce pain, inflammation, and fever by blocking certain enzymes in the body. Nurses often administer NSAIDs to patients to help manage conditions such as arthritis, muscle pain, and headaches. It is important for nurses to understand the appropriate use, dosages, side effects, and contraindications of NSAIDs when caring for patients.

NSAIDs are a commonly used class of medications in nursing practice due to their effectiveness in managing pain and inflammation. Nurses play a crucial role in administering NSAIDs to patients, monitoring their response to the medication, and educating them about potential side effects and interactions.

Some commonly used NSAIDs include ibuprofen, naproxen, and aspirin. These medications can be available over the counter or by prescription, depending on the strength and formulation. Nurses need to assess patients for allergies, medical history, and concurrent medications that may interact with NSAIDs before administering them.

In nursing practice, NSAIDs are often used to manage conditions like osteoarthritis, rheumatoid arthritis, menstrual cramps, and mild to moderate pain. Nurses need to closely monitor patients for adverse reactions such as gastrointestinal ulcers, kidney dysfunction, and cardiovascular effects, especially in long-term or high-dose NSAID use.

Patient education is vital when administering NSAIDs. Nurses should inform patients about proper dosing, potential side effects, and the importance of taking NSAIDs with food to reduce gastrointestinal irritation. It is also crucial for nurses to emphasize the importance of not exceeding the recommended dose and to seek medical attention if they experience any concerning symptoms.

In summary, NSAIDs are important medications in nursing practice for managing pain and inflammation in patients. Nurses play a key role in safely administering NSAIDs, monitoring patients for adverse effects, and educating them about the proper use of these medications.

274. Omentum

The omentum is a fold of peritoneum that connects the stomach with other abdominal organs. It consists of two parts: the greater omentum and the lesser omentum. In nursing, understanding the structure and function of the omentum is important when assessing and caring for patients with abdominal issues or surgeries.

The greater omentum is a large, apron-like structure that hangs down from the greater curvature of the stomach and covers the intestines. It plays a role in immune responses and can help isolate areas of infection or injury within the abdominal cavity. The lesser omentum, on the other hand, connects the lesser curvature of the stomach and the proximal part of the duodenum to the liver.

In nursing, knowledge of the Omentum is crucial to assess patients with abdominal pain, inflammation, or other related issues. Nurses need to understand the potential implications of omental involvement in various health conditions, such as peritonitis, abdominal trauma, or abdominal surgeries. Communication and collaboration with other healthcare professionals are essential to provide comprehensive care for patients with omental-related concerns.

By staying informed about the anatomy and function of the omentum, nurses can contribute effectively to the assessment, planning, and implementation of care for patients with abdominal conditions involving this important structure.

275. Ophthalmologist

An ophthalmologist is a medical doctor who specializes in the diagnosis and treatment of eye diseases and disorders. They perform eye exams, prescribe corrective lenses, diagnose eye conditions, perform surgeries, and manage various eye conditions such as cataracts, glaucoma, macular degeneration, and more. Ophthalmologists are not nurses; they are physicians who have completed medical school and specialized training in ophthalmology.

Ophthalmologists undergo extensive training to become experts in the field of eye care. After completing medical school, they typically undergo a residency program that focuses on ophthalmology. During this training, they learn to diagnose and manage a wide range of eye conditions, perform surgeries such as cataract surgery, LASIK procedures, and more complex interventions.

Ophthalmologists work closely with other healthcare professionals, including nurses, optometrists, and opticians, to provide comprehensive eye care to patients of all ages. They play a crucial role in preserving and improving vision, as well as managing chronic eye conditions to prevent further complications.

In summary, ophthalmologists are highly specialized medical professionals who focus on the diagnosis and treatment of eye diseases and disorders. Their expertise is essential in ensuring the health and well-being of patients with various eye conditions.

276. Osteoporosis

Osteoporosis is a medical condition characterized by a decrease in bone density and quality, leading to an increased risk of fractures. In nursing, understanding osteoporosis is essential as nurses play a crucial role in educating patients about prevention, managing medications to help prevent fractures, and providing support and care to those affected by the condition. Nurses may be involved in assessing patients for risk factors, implementing prevention strategies, and promoting bone health through patient education and medication management.

Nurses caring for patients with osteoporosis also play a vital role in developing individualized care plans to help manage the condition effectively. This may involve collaborating with other healthcare professionals, such as physicians, physical therapists, and dietitians, to provide comprehensive care. Nurses need to educate patients about lifestyle modifications, such as regular weight-bearing exercises, adequate calcium and vitamin D intake, and falls prevention strategies to minimize the risk of fractures. Moreover, they assist in monitoring the effectiveness of treatment plans, managing complications of osteoporosis, and providing emotional support to patients coping with the challenges of living with the condition.

In summary, understanding osteoporosis and its implications in nursing involves a holistic approach to patient care that encompasses prevention, education, management, and support. By staying informed about the latest research and best practices in osteoporosis care, nurses can make a significant impact on improving the quality of life for individuals affected by this prevalent bone disease.

277. Oxygen therapy

Oxygen therapy in nursing refers to the administration of oxygen as a medical intervention to individuals who have difficulty breathing or who are not getting enough oxygen into their bloodstream. This treatment is commonly used for patients with conditions such as pneumonia, chronic obstructive pulmonary disease (COPD), or respiratory distress. Oxygen therapy helps to increase the oxygen levels in the blood, making it easier for the body to function properly. Nurses play a crucial role in assessing the need for oxygen therapy, monitoring patients during treatment, and ensuring that the therapy is administered safely and effectively.

278. Pap smear

A Pap smear, also known as a Pap test, is a screening procedure used to detect abnormal cervical cells, which may indicate the presence of cervical cancer or pre-cancerous conditions. During a Pap smear, a healthcare provider collects cells from the cervix (the lower part of the uterus that connects to the vagina) and sends them to a laboratory for examination under a microscope. This test is important for early detection and prevention of cervical cancer. Nurses may assist with performing Pap smears and educating patients about the procedure and its importance.

279. Paraplegia

Paraplegia is a condition characterized by the loss of motor and sensory function in the lower part of the body, typically due to spinal cord injury or disease. In nursing, care for individuals with paraplegia involves assisting with activities of daily living, monitoring for complications such as pressure ulcers or urinary tract infections, providing education on injury prevention and management, and offering emotional support to help cope with the challenges of living with a spinal cord injury. Nurses may also assist with rehabilitation programs designed to improve mobility and independence for individuals with paraplegia.

280. Parkinson's disease

Parkinson's disease is a progressive nervous system disorder that affects movement. It is characterized by tremors, stiffness, slowness of movement, and difficulty with balance and coordination. In the context of nursing, understanding Parkinson's disease involves recognizing its symptoms, providing appropriate care to manage those symptoms, educating patients and their families about the condition, and supporting the individual in maintaining their quality of life. Nursing care for individuals with Parkinson's disease may involve medication management, physical therapy, emotional support, and assistance with activities of daily living. Care plans are tailored to meet the specific needs of each patient and to promote their overall well-being.

281. Paronychia

Paronychia is a common infection that occurs around the fingernails or toenails. It can be caused by bacteria, fungi, or yeast entering the skin around the nail, often due to factors such as injury, biting nails, manicures, or frequent hand washing. In nursing, paronychia would be a condition that nurses may encounter and provide care for, typically involving treatment such as warm water soaks, proper wound care, possible drainage of pus, and, if necessary, prescribing antibiotics. It's important to address paronychia promptly to prevent complications and promote healing.

282. Peak flow

"Peak flow" in nursing refers to a measurement used to assess how well a person's lungs are working. It measures the maximum rate at which a person can push air out of their lungs. Peak flow measurements are often used to monitor and manage conditions such as asthma or other respiratory diseases. By tracking peak flow readings over time, healthcare providers can assess lung function, adjust treatment plans, and identify potential flare-ups or worsening of respiratory symptoms.

283. Perfusion

Perfusion in nursing refers to the process of delivering blood to a capillary bed in tissues. It ensures the delivery of oxygen and nutrients to cells and the removal of waste products. Adequate perfusion is vital for normal organ function. Nurses often monitor perfusion by assessing vital signs, skin color, capillary refill time, and other indicators to ensure that organs are receiving proper blood flow. Impaired perfusion can lead to serious health issues and organ damage.

284. Perineal

The term "perineal" in nursing refers to the region between the anus and the external genitalia. This area is often the focus of care for patients in various healthcare settings, especially those who have undergone certain medical procedures or women who have given birth. Perineal care involves cleaning, monitoring, and maintaining the health of this area to prevent infections and other complications.

Perineal care is an important aspect of nursing hygiene and patient comfort. It involves regular cleaning and inspection of the perineal area to prevent infections and promote healing, especially after childbirth, surgery, or for patients with incontinence issues. Proper perineal care helps to maintain skin integrity, prevent irritation, and reduce the risk of urinary tract infections or other complications.

Nurses must be knowledgeable about the proper techniques for perineal care, including using gentle cleansing methods, avoiding harsh soaps or products that may cause irritation, and ensuring thorough but gentle drying of the area. Additionally, nurses must be sensitive to patients' privacy and comfort during perineal care procedures, maintaining professionalism and respecting the individual's dignity throughout the process.
By providing effective perineal care, nurses play a crucial role in promoting patients' overall well-being and preventing potential complications that could arise from poor hygiene practices in the perineal area.

285. Peritoneum

The peritoneum is a large, thin membrane that lines the abdominal cavity and covers the abdominal organs. It plays an essential role in providing protection and support to the abdominal organs as well as in the secretion and absorption of fluids within the abdominal cavity. In nursing, an understanding of the peritoneum and its function is important in assessing and managing patients with abdominal conditions or disorders.

The peritoneum is composed of two layers: the parietal peritoneum, which lines the abdominal wall, and the visceral peritoneum, which covers the abdominal organs. Between these two layers is a potential space called the peritoneal cavity, which contains a small amount of fluid that helps reduce friction between the organs as they move within the abdominal cavity.

In nursing practice, understanding the anatomy and function of the peritoneum is crucial in assessing patients with abdominal pain, distension, or other symptoms related to abdominal organs. Nurses may need to perform physical assessments, including palpation and percussion of the abdomen, to detect any abnormalities in the peritoneal area. They may also need to monitor patients for signs of peritonitis, which is inflammation of the peritoneum often caused by infection or injury.

Additionally, nurses may be involved in procedures such as paracentesis, which involves removing fluid from the peritoneal cavity for diagnostic or therapeutic purposes. By having a thorough knowledge of the peritoneum and its significance in abdominal health, nurses can provide effective care and support to patients with abdominal conditions.

286. Phototherapy

Phototherapy in nursing refers to a treatment method that uses specific wavelengths of light to address various health conditions. In neonatal nursing, phototherapy is commonly used to treat jaundice in newborns. The light helps break down the excess bilirubin in the baby's blood, which is causing the yellow discoloration of the skin and eyes. Nurses monitor the baby's response to phototherapy and make adjustments as needed to ensure proper treatment and manage potential side effects.

287. Placenta

In nursing, the term "placenta" refers to an organ that develops in the uterus during pregnancy. It provides oxygen and nutrients to the fetus, removes waste products from the fetus, and produces hormones to support pregnancy. After the baby is born, the placenta is expelled from the mother's body during the third stage of labor. Nursing care related to the placenta includes monitoring its delivery, ensuring its complete expulsion, and assessing for any signs of complications such as retained placenta or postpartum hemorrhage.

288. Pneumothorax

Pneumothorax in nursing is a condition characterized by the presence of air or gas in the pleural cavity, which is the space between the lungs and the chest wall. This accumulation of air can cause the lung to collapse partially or completely, leading to symptoms such as chest pain, shortness of breath, and in severe cases, respiratory distress. Nursing care for a patient with pneumothorax includes monitoring the patient's respiratory status, providing oxygen therapy as needed, assisting with chest tube placement if necessary, and assessing for any complications.

289. Polyps

"Polyps" in nursing refer to abnormal tissue growths that can occur in various parts of the body, such as the colon, nose, uterus, or vocal cords. Polyps can be noncancerous (benign) or in some cases, they can be precancerous or cancerous. The presence of polyps may require monitoring, removal, or further investigation depending on the location and type of polyp. In nursing, understanding the implications of polyps and providing appropriate care and education to patients is essential.

290. Postoperative

Postoperative nursing refers to the period of care and recovery that occurs after a surgical procedure has been performed on a patient. During the postoperative phase, nurses are responsible for closely monitoring the patient's vital signs, managing pain, preventing complications, and assisting with the patient's transition to recovery. Nurses play a crucial role in ensuring that patients receive the appropriate care and support they need after surgery to promote healing and overall well-being.

291. Prosthesis

Prosthesis in nursing refers to an artificial device that replaces a missing body part. This can include prosthetic limbs, such as arms or legs, prosthetic joints, or prosthetic teeth. Nurses may be involved in helping patients adjust to and care for their prosthetic devices. Prostheses are designed to improve the function and quality of life for individuals who have experienced an amputation or loss of a body part.

292. Ptosis

Ptosis in nursing refers to the drooping of the upper eyelid, which can be due to various reasons such as muscle weakness, nerve damage, or injury. It can affect one or both eyes and may impair vision depending on the severity. Nurses may encounter patients with ptosis in clinical settings and should be able to recognize the condition and provide appropriate care or referral to a healthcare provider.

The drooping of the upper eyelid in ptosis may vary in severity, with some cases causing minimal obstruction of vision while others can significantly impact a person's ability to see clearly. Patients with ptosis may experience symptoms such as eye fatigue, difficulty keeping the affected eye open, and compensatory actions like raising their eyebrows to lift the eyelid. In nursing, recognizing ptosis can be important for assessing the patient's overall eye health and determining if further evaluation or intervention is needed by an ophthalmologist or other healthcare provider. Nurses can also provide education to patients about the condition, potential causes, and available treatment options.

293. Quadriplegia

Quadriplegia is a condition in which a person experiences paralysis in all four limbs, typically due to spinal cord injury or illness. In nursing, caring for patients with quadriplegia involves addressing their unique needs, providing assistance with activities of daily living, monitoring for complications such as pressure ulcers, and promoting rehabilitation and independence to the extent possible. It requires a comprehensive and holistic approach to ensure the well-being and quality of life of individuals with quadriplegia education on how to manage their condition and adapt to their limitations. Nurses also play a vital role in advocating for patients with quadriplegia, ensuring that they have access to necessary resources, support services, and rehabilitation programs that can help improve their quality of life.

In addition to physical care, nurses also provide emotional support to patients with quadriplegia and their families, as adjusting to a life-changing condition like quadriplegia can be emotionally challenging for everyone involved. Nurses help patients cope with feelings of frustration, sadness, and loss, and provide reassurance and encouragement as they navigate their new reality.

Nurses working with patients with quadriplegia must be knowledgeable about assistive devices, mobility aids, and techniques to help improve patients' independence and function. They work closely with a multidisciplinary team that may include physical therapists, occupational therapists, social workers, and physicians to develop individualized care plans tailored to each patient's specific needs and goals.

Overall, nursing care for individuals with quadriplegia is focused on promoting optimal physical, emotional, and social well-being, empowering patients to lead fulfilling lives to the best of their abilities despite their physical limitations. It requires compassion, empathy, expertise, and a willingness to go above and beyond to support patients in their journey towards recovery and adaptation to life with quadriplegia.

294. Reflexes

Reflexes in nursing refer to involuntary responses by the body to certain stimuli. Nurses often assess reflexes as part of a physical examination to evaluate the functioning of the nervous system. Common reflexes tested include the knee-jerk reflex, pupillary reflex, and reflexes in response to light touch or other stimuli. Abnormal reflexes can provide important diagnostic information about neurologic functioning and potential health issues.

Reflexes are essential for maintaining the body's normal function and protecting it from harm. They are controlled by the nervous system and occur rapidly, often without conscious thought. In nursing, assessing reflexes can help healthcare providers identify neurological disorders, spinal cord injuries, and other conditions affecting the nervous system.

There are different types of reflexes that nurses may test during a physical examination. Some common reflexes include:

1. **Deep tendon reflexes**: These reflexes involve striking a tendon with a reflex hammer to evoke a muscle contraction. The patellar reflex (knee-jerk reflex) is a well-known example of a deep tendon reflex.

2. **Superficial reflexes**: These reflexes involve stimulation of the skin to elicit a response. Examples include the plantar reflex (Babinski reflex), which involves stroking the sole of the foot to observe the response of the toes.

3. **Autonomic reflexes**: These reflexes control activities of the internal organs, such as heart rate, digestion, and blood pressure regulation. Examples include the pupillary reflex, which controls the constriction and dilation of the pupils in response to light.

Nurses use their assessment of reflexes, along with other physical examination findings, patient history, and diagnostic tests, to formulate a comprehensive care plan for their patients. In cases where abnormal reflexes are detected, further evaluation and intervention may be necessary to address any underlying health issues. By understanding and interpreting reflex responses, nurses play a crucial role in promoting patient well-being and overall health.

295. Regurgitation

Regurgitation in nursing refers to the condition were food, liquid, or stomach contents flow back up from the stomach into the esophagus or even into the mouth. This can happen due to various reasons such as GERD (gastroesophageal reflux disease), a weak lower esophageal sphincter, or other digestive issues. Regurgitation can cause discomfort and other symptoms, and it is important for healthcare providers to assess and address it appropriately to provide relief and prevent complications.

Regurgitation in nursing is a common symptom that nurses may encounter when assessing patients with gastrointestinal issues. It can manifest as the involuntary return of ingested food, liquid, or stomach contents back up the esophagus, leading to a sensation of fluid coming up into the throat or mouth. Patients may experience regurgitation as a result of conditions such as GERD, hiatal hernia, esophageal motility disorders, or anatomical abnormalities of the upper gastrointestinal tract.

Nurses play a crucial role in assessing and managing regurgitation in patients. They may need to collect a detailed medical history, perform a physical examination, and possibly recommend diagnostic tests such as an upper endoscopy or esophageal pH monitoring to determine the underlying cause of the regurgitation. Nursing interventions for regurgitation may include lifestyle modifications (e.g., diet changes, weight loss), medications to reduce stomach acid production or improve esophageal motility, and patient education on symptom management and prevention.

Effective communication with the healthcare team and the patient is essential in providing holistic care for individuals experiencing regurgitation. Nurses should collaborate with physicians, dietitians, and other healthcare professionals to develop a comprehensive care plan tailored to the patient's specific needs and goals. By addressing the underlying cause of regurgitation and implementing appropriate interventions, nurses can help improve patient outcomes and quality of life.

296. Rhonchi

Rhonchi in nursing refers to a type of abnormal breath sound that can be heard upon auscultation of the lungs. These sounds are often described as continuous, low-pitched, rattling, or snoring sounds that can be heard during inspiration and expiration. Rhonchi are often associated with airway secretions or mucus in the larger airways of the lungs and may indicate conditions such as bronchitis, pneumonia, or chronic obstructive pulmonary disease (COPD). Monitoring and assessing for the presence of rhonchi is an important part of a comprehensive respiratory assessment in nursing practice.

297. Serotonin

Serotonin is a neurotransmitter that plays a crucial role in the regulation of mood, sleep, appetite, and other physiological functions in the body. In nursing, understanding serotonin and its functions is important because imbalances or deficiencies in this neurotransmitter can contribute to various mental health disorders such as depression, anxiety, and mood disorders. Nurses may encounter patients with conditions related to serotonin levels and may need to provide care and support to help manage these conditions.

298. Sickle cell anemia

Sickle cell anemia is a genetic blood disorder that affects the red blood cells. In sickle cell anemia, the red blood cells become rigid, sticky, and sickle-shaped, leading to various complications such as pain, anemia, organ damage, and increased risk of infections. Nurses play a crucial role in managing and caring for patients with sickle cell anemia by providing supportive care, monitoring symptoms, administering treatments, and educating patients and their families about the condition.

Sickle cell anemia is caused by a mutation in the gene that produces hemoglobin, the protein responsible for carrying oxygen in red blood cells. This genetic mutation results in the production of abnormal hemoglobin known as hemoglobin S, which causes the red blood cells to become rigid and form a characteristic sickle shape under certain conditions, such as low oxygen levels or dehydration.

The sickle-shaped red blood cells are not as flexible as normal red blood cells, making it difficult for them to pass through small blood vessels. This can lead to blockages in the blood vessels, causing tissue damage and pain. Individuals with sickle cell anemia experience episodes of pain known as sickle cell crises, which can vary in severity and duration.

In addition to pain crises, individuals with sickle cell anemia are also at increased risk of developing complications such as acute chest syndrome, stroke, infections, and organ damage. Management of sickle cell anemia includes treatments to reduce pain, prevent complications, and manage symptoms, as well as measures to promote overall health and well-being.

Nurses caring for patients with sickle cell anemia play a vital role in assessing and monitoring their condition, providing supportive care, managing pain and complications, administering medications, and educating patients and their families about the disease. By working collaboratively with a healthcare team, nurses can help improve the quality of life for individuals living with sickle cell anemia.

299. Stasis

Stasis in nursing typically refers to a condition where there is a lack of movement or flow of bodily fluids in a particular area of the body. This can be related to blood stasis, where there is a lack of proper circulation leading to pooling of blood in a specific area, often seen in conditions like deep vein thrombosis. Nurses may address stasis by implementing measures to improve circulation and prevent complications such as blood clots or pressure ulcers.

As a result, the affected area may become swollen, discolored, and painful. In the context of nursing, managing stasis involves promoting circulation through strategies such as encouraging movement and positioning changes, providing compression therapy, administering medications to prevent blood clots, and monitoring for signs of complications. Nurses play a crucial role in assessing patients for signs of stasis and implementing interventions to prevent its negative consequences. By addressing stasis promptly and effectively, nurses can help prevent complications and promote better outcomes for their patients.

300. Tonicity

Tonicity in nursing refers to the relative concentration of solutes in two fluids separated by a semipermeable membrane. It describes how a solution can affect the movement of water across a cell membrane. Tonicity is important in situations like intravenous fluid administration or wound management, where the right balance of solutes is necessary to prevent dehydration or tissue damage. There are three main types of tonicity: isotonic, hypotonic, and hypertonic solutions, each of which has different effects on cells and tissues.

Tonicity plays a crucial role in maintaining the balance of fluids in the body and ensuring proper cell function. Understanding tonicity is essential for healthcare providers, especially in fields like nursing, where they may need to administer intravenous fluids or irrigate wounds with the right type of solution.

Isotonic solutions have the same concentration of solutes as human blood and cells. When an isotonic solution is administered intravenously, it helps maintain the normal osmotic pressure of the blood and prevents cells from shrinking or swelling.

Hypotonic solutions have a lower concentration of solutes compared to human blood. When a hypotonic solution is used, water moves into the cells by osmosis, causing them to swell. Hypotonic solutions are sometimes used to rehydrate patients who are dehydrated.

Hypertonic solutions, on the other hand, have a higher concentration of solutes than human blood. When a hypertonic solution is administered, water moves out of the cells, causing them to shrink. Hypertonic solutions are used to draw excess fluid out of tissues or cells, such as in the case of cerebral edema.

Nurses must assess the patient's condition and select the appropriate tonicity of solutions to ensure safe and effective treatment. Monitoring the patient's response to the solution is crucial to prevent complications related to tonicity, such as fluid overload or dehydration.